SEX EDUCATION FOR BOYS
A PARENT'S GUIDE

SEX
EDUCATION
FOR BOYS
A Parent's
Guide

Practical Advice on Puberty, Sex, and Relationships

Scott Todnem

R

**ROCKRIDGE
PRESS**

For general information on our other products and services or to obtain technical support, please contact our Customer Care Department within the United States at (866) 744-2665, or outside the United States at (510) 253-0500.

Rockridge Press publishes its books in a variety of electronic and print formats. Some content that appears in print may not be available in electronic books, and vice versa.

Interior and Cover Designer: Jill Lee
Art Producer: Melissa Malinowsky
Editor: Carolyn Abate
Production Editor: Matthew Burnett
Production Manager: David Zapanta

Illustration © Conor Buckley, p. 11
Author photograph courtesy of Ashley Summers

Paperback ISBN: 978-1-63807-709-1
eBook ISBN: 978-1-63807-543-1

R0

This book could not have been possible without my own parents, Guy and Nancy, who nurtured me through the ups and downs of adolescence by creating space to question, to learn, and to love life. I am also in unending awe of my wife, Sarah, for being my calm, my constant, and my partner in parenthood.

CONTENTS

Introduction *ix*

How to Talk to Your Son about Sex *xii*

PART I
WHEN BOYS GROW UP 2

Chapter One: A Puberty Primer 5

Chapter Two: What It Means to Be a "Man" 16

Chapter Three: Gender, Sex, and Sexual Health 33

PART II
FOUNDATIONAL PARENTING STRATEGIES 48

Chapter Four: Defining and Sharing Your Values 51

Chapter Five: Establishing Mutual Trust and Respect 57

Chapter Six: Facilitating Openness 63

Chapter Seven: Embracing Vulnerability 69

Chapter Eight: Encouraging Emotional Intimacy 75

PART III
SPECIFIC SEXUAL HEALTH STRATEGIES FOR BOYS 82

Chapter Nine: Nurturing Healthy
Dating Relationships 85

Chapter Ten: Instilling a Comprehensive
Understanding of Consent 91

Chapter Eleven: Exploring Safer Sex 98

Chapter Twelve: Challenging the Expectations
of the Internet and Porn 104

Chapter Thirteen: Discussing Texting
and Social Media 110

Chapter Fourteen: Raising an Ally 116

PART IV
FREQUENTLY ASKED QUESTIONS, ANSWERED 122

Resources 136

References 138

Index 142

INTRODUCTION

Remember the beginning of parenthood? The start of your caregiving role? However and whenever you entered the fold—birth, adoption, blended family; infancy, toddler years, elementary school—it was a whirlwind of responsibility. Not to mention the questions! "Why is the sky blue?" "Where does bathwater go?" "Where do babies come from?"

As kids age, the subject matter changes and the questions might be redirected, but our teens and preteens still wonder. And with bigger bodies and bigger brains come bigger topics. Adolescents want to know how the world works and what is normal, but these are often coded questions about puberty, sex, relationships, and more.

Consider this: When we have a talk, *the* talk, with our kids, and believe our work is done, we've simply put the topic of puberty and sex at arm's length. We have placed it "over there" so we, the adults, can move on with our lives. But when we create an environment where questions are the norm and conversations can continue, our children can feel safe to come to us for understanding. Isn't that our real job anyway? This book is for the parents who have decided that arm's length is not good enough. This is for the parents who want to keep the lines of communication open.

When it comes to discussing sexuality with your son, no one knows your child the way you do. But within the pages of this book, we can empower you with facts, concepts, and counsel so you can decide on the best ways to support your child's specific needs as he navigates the challenges ahead.

In PART I you'll find a general overview of the puberty transition into adulthood, specifically as it relates to boys, their relationships, and sexual health. These chapters will clarify terminology for the remainder of the book and serve as a review of what adolescent boys undergo physically, mentally, emotionally, and socially. This will help answer questions and correct misconceptions about the realities of puberty.

Throughout PART II, we'll explore some general strategies to help parents connect and care for adolescents. The goal here is to provide guidance that allows parents to align evolving societal standards with their values. Topics covered include fostering conversations, building trust, and encouraging comfort with vulnerability and emotional intimacy.

With PART III, we'll dive into specific parenting strategies related to sexual wellness. This section will challenge caregivers to be progressive in their thoughts and actions. We'll equip you to support adolescent boys through issues such as gender identity, sexuality, consent, safe sex, pornography, and being a considerate ally to others.

And in PART IV, we'll conclude with a roster of 25 frequently asked questions, and answers, specific to boys and sexual wellness.

If the prospect of discussing these subjects with your son makes you feel anxious or uncomfortable, that's normal. These are delicate issues, and of course you want to get it right for your child's sake. I know just how you feel. As an author, speaker, and health education teacher I have the luxury of experience. I have the privilege of years and years of giving the talk—many talks—to teens. And yet at times I'm still unsure of myself. I'm still nervous or uncomfortable. I'm still worried about saying the right things.

But I've seen for myself how important these conversations can be. I'm a parent of four amazing kids who sing and scream and laugh and cry. In our household, we try to follow a body-positive, factual, respectful approach to relationships and sexuality. We maintain that sexual wellness includes physical, mental, emotional, and social health in close connection with safe, pleasurable experiences that are free of coercion, discrimination, and violence. My hope is that this book will lay that same foundation for you and your family.

HOW TO TALK TO YOUR SON ABOUT SEX

You may have serious trepidation about discussing sexual issues with your son. Or maybe you are eager to engage and educate. Perhaps you fall somewhere in between. Wherever your comfort level, know that it's okay. In the end, as long as you exhibit care and concern for their well-being, adolescents will notice and benefit from your involvement. My advice is to worry less about doing the wrong thing and worry more about doing *something*. Even when you don't have the right words or the right answers, make sure you are there for your son. This book will provide concrete examples of how to do that.

Whatever fumbles and flubs you make—and we all make them—your unique path as a parent will run true if you ask these questions along the way:

- ▶ Am I doing my best to use accurate language and terminology?
- ▶ Am I being genuine and remaining positive?
- ▶ Am I modeling lifelong learning and other healthy behavior?

Empowering you to answer "yes" to those questions is the core objective of this book. We'll be referencing all three of those concepts throughout these chapters, together.

The Challenges of Talking to Your Son about Sex

Great news: You don't need to be an expert in anatomy, psychology, or sociology to initiate conversations with your son about sex. Try your best to understand current social trends and to use correct, accurate terminology in your conversations.

Talking about sex is challenging enough without muddying the waters with imprecise language. Using the proper terms will help with clarity. And it will help you both become comfortable in having adult conversations that are frank and free of euphemisms. You'll find vocabulary and terminology throughout this book that you can use with confidence; here are some key terms and their definitions to keep in mind:

Sexual wellness is a factual, respectful approach to sexuality and sexual relationships. It includes physical, mental, emotional, and social health, in close connection with safe, pleasurable sexual experiences that are free of coercion, discrimination, and violence.

Puberty is the physical change a person undergoes as they develop from a child into an adult.

Adolescence is the time between the beginning of puberty and the start of adulthood.

Male and related terms (masculine, boy, man, guy), as well as pronouns like he, his, and him, appear throughout this book. They may not fit everyone's identity, expression, or preferred way of speech, but they're intended as general terms.

Though the phrases *male reproductive system* and *female reproductive system* may sound scientific, a more accurate wording is to discuss what happens for "a person with testicles," or "a person with ovaries," aka "penis owners" or "uterus owners." Other options include the terms "assigned male gender" and "assigned female gender." If you're new to it, this kind of language can feel a bit clunky at first. But separating the definition of "male" and "female" from the presence of certain glands and organs is a more precise way of describing what goes on during puberty. It also allows us to encompass a large audience that has children of varying bodies and backgrounds.

Sex as a reference to one's anatomy is a biological concept based on appearance of genitalia and other reproductive organs.

Gender is a social construct that describes characteristics such as behavior, roles, and relationships and how those attributes are expressed.

LGBTQIA+ stands for lesbian, gay, bisexual, transgender, queer/ questioning, intersex, asexual, and more.

Sexual contact is the deliberate touching of a person's intimate body parts, including lips, genitalia, breasts, anus, buttocks, or clothing covering any of those areas. It can also be any touch that is considered erotic, on any part of the body.

As you think about deploying these terms in conversation with your child, keep these points in mind:

Take the reins. For the majority of discussions with adolescents, it's adults who lead. Some boys may instigate conversations with a quick question here or there, but for the most part the process needs to start with you.

Don't wait. Start age-appropriate conversations about growth and sexuality early and often, even before you suspect your son has hit any puberty milestones or has become sexually active. If he's an older teen and you're just getting around to this, you're not too late! Start things up right away with short bursts of info and insight.

Yeah, it's cringy. Truth be told, you can expect a bit of awkwardness. It's unrealistic to expect perfect "heart-to-heart" talks like we sometimes see in movies or TV shows. Refrain from trying to ease your discomfort by using too many metaphors, idioms, or cute sayings. A straightforward approach is effective and generally welcomed by teens. Treat your son as the young adult he is, and you'll notice respect is returned.

Avoid this phrase. One specific idiom to consider staying away from is referring to sex or any related talk as "the birds and the bees." Unless you'd like to use sarcasm as an icebreaker, this reference is antiquated and even confusing. If you've already used similar phrases, no worries—simply use human terminology going forward!

To further inform your conversations, you'll find example dialogue throughout parts II and III of this book.

The Importance of Positivity

Along with your choice of words—employing the correct and accurate terminology—your choice of attitude also plays a huge role in giving your son the support and guidance he needs. Although cautions and warnings have their place, your goal is not to frighten or intimidate your child into staying out of trouble. Rather, you should strive for a positive tone that portrays a genuine, ongoing optimism about your son's growth and development. Three concepts will help you stay positive in the most challenging conversations—and be a model of compassion and empathy for your son to follow.

Positive body image. This includes your son's view of, and feelings about, himself. What does your son see when he looks in the mirror? What does he think his body is capable of, and how does he feel about that?

Body positivity. Body positivity is the notion that all human bodies have worth, regardless of physical ability, race, or gender.

It calls for treating other people's bodies with kindness and celebration, particularly those body types that have historically been marginalized.

Sex positivity. A sex-positive mindset involves recognizing and promoting sexuality as a natural, healthy, pleasurable part of any human experience. It's essential for comprehensive sex education. Sex positivity encourages your child to explore their gender and sexuality without shame or fear of judgment. It gives them permission to find out who they are, what they like, and what works for them by affirming their personal values and beliefs without oppressing the sexuality of others.

It's important to know that sex positivity doesn't insist on promiscuity, nudism, or other similar concepts. It can hold a place for those activities, so long as they're consensual for everyone involved. However, sex positivity doesn't condone inappropriate or nonconsensual behavior, or infringing on others' rights in any way.

Human sexuality is sometimes explained as or assumed to be dirty, disgusting, and/or dangerous. Although specific cases of sexual contact might prove to be risky or even harmful, sex is not necessarily naughty. Sex is not inherently bad.

Let's repeat that so it sinks in: Sex is not inherently bad.

Initiating Conversations

Now that we've discussed the quality of the conversations you'll be having with your child, let's get practical and explore just how to get these wonderfully positive discussions started. Even if you and your son had a "we can talk about anything" kind of relationship until now, puberty can bring some hesitation to the table—for both of you. So try these strategies for initiating and maintaining quality conversations about puberty, relationships, and sexual wellness.

Be the catalyst. Remember, not all communication on relationships and sex will stem from your son. Saying "I'm here if you need anything" feels right, but that can be more of a closed door than one might think. Start discussions yourself by directly addressing whatever you'd like to chat about.

Maintain relationship boundaries. Don't try to seem young by tossing out slang that you think is current. Don't pretend to know it all, and definitely don't try to be your son's friend. Boys want and need a parent, plain and simple.

Be specific. Avoid generalizations like "Be safe tonight—you know what I mean?" If you want to talk about condoms, then talk about condoms. That goes for any topic, of course, from more innocuous items like hygiene to much trickier issues like pornography.

Be patient. Try to keep in mind that although you have already been through puberty—and survived—your son has not. You may be reviewing this information for the second, third, or hundredth time. This is probably his first time hearing it. Even if it isn't, you'll likely have to go over it many times before it takes hold.

Try talking shoulder to shoulder. When sitting across the table, face-to-face with an authority figure, adolescent boys may feel confronted, defensive, or embarrassed. With sexual wellness, putting your son at ease is more imperative. Try chatting while you're sitting on the couch, watching a slow game or a movie you've both seen before. Or use the car! A short trip, while you're running an errand or ferrying him to a friend's house, is a great opportunity for a dialogue. You're both facing the road, he can't run away, and there's an end point in sight if the ride gets bumpy.

Be yourself. Avoid trying to be cooler, stricter, or otherwise different; be the same parent you've always been. Stay away from saying or doing something just because you *think* you should, especially if you're not feeling it. That includes recommendations you find in this book: Make sure everything gels with your parenting style so you can match your message to your comfort level and personality strengths.

Fielding Questions

According to cinematic stereotypes, we parents should dread questions from our children about sexual wellness. But in reality, questions are exactly what we want. As caregivers, we want our sons to come to us for answers just as often, if not more so, than they turn to friends, older siblings, or the internet.

You can't anticipate every single question your son will ask you, but by the time you finish this book you'll definitely have a larger knowledge base to draw on for answers. In the meantime, here are a few general principles to rely on when fielding queries about sex and relationships:

Brevity is a virtue. Keep things short! Avoid long-winded discussions that are particularly one-sided on your end. Err on the "less is more" philosophy; you can always follow up at a later time.

If you don't know . . . then say you don't know. No one is an expert on everything. Get comfortable with this phrase: "I don't know, but I will do my best to find out." Use that quote often and unapologetically. If it makes sense, you can do the research together. Use this book's Resources section as a starting point.

To err is human. And to care is humane. If—when—mistakes come up, acknowledge them and make a correction if possible. Try saying, "I made a mistake. Sorry, I'm still learning things, too." This is vital for showing your son what lifelong learning looks like.

Buy yourself some time. If you need more time to answer questions than what's available at the moment, simply state the truth. "Great question. I need a little time before I can give that topic the attention it deserves. Let's talk at _____. Sound good?" Caveat: Be absolutely certain you do circle back. Write a note, set an alarm as a reminder, or do whatever you need to make sure you don't miss the time you promised your son.

One thing at a time. Puberty and sexuality are complex topics. You don't have to hit all the talking points at once. Nor should you; multiple conversations throughout months and years of adolescence are the most effective method. If there are several parts to a question, it's okay to tackle the most pressing issue first and table the others.

Remain honest. Avoid withholding information because you're concerned it will be used in a negative way. There is no research— none—to support that the rate of sexual contact among teens increases because of sex education. Teens aren't "doing it" (pardon the euphemism) because we talk about it with them. In contrast, healthy relationship behavior—making sure sexual behavior is consensual, protected, and pleasurable—*does* increase with conversation.

Express gratitude. Quite possibly, it took your son a lot of nerve to come to you with a question. A simple appreciation, like "Thanks for coming to me," goes a long way toward keeping the dialogue doors open.

How This Book Can Help

Sometimes talking with teens about puberty, relationships, and sex feels a little like a test of your parenting abilities. Thankfully it's an open-book test, and you're free to double-check your answers any time you need to. Use this book to plan and prep for the challenging, and rewarding, times ahead. And return to it for specific advice when a particular difficulty arises.

If you haven't started discussing sexual health matters with your son, you'll find that part I of this book will give you a good grounding in the physical and other changes that come with puberty. With the facts and figures in hand, you'll feel confident and ready to open that dialogue.

If you're feeling overwhelmed by the prospect of parenting an adolescent, in part II we'll share some foundational approaches and additional ideas for parenting through your son's sexual education. You'll find case studies of parenting scenarios and sample dialogues to help you put best practices into action.

If helping your son navigate the sexual storm of puberty is your most immediate parenting concern at the moment, part III is the compass you need. In these chapters, the case studies, guidelines, and dialogues will equip you with specific strategies for dealing with the complexities of sexual health.

And finally, when you need to quickly drill down to specifics, part IV's collection of frequently asked questions will help you and your son tackle some of the most common sexual health issues that you're likely to face.

Feeling any test anxiety yet? No need. Always remember: You got this.

PART I

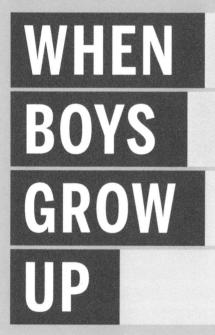

WHEN
BOYS
GROW
UP

Our first task together is to provide a holistic overview of a boy's transition into adulthood, while previewing concepts related to sexual health and development. Think of part I as a baseline of knowledge and language that will support the more nuanced conversations you'll have during your son's formative years. In these chapters we'll review physical development through puberty, what boys tend to be concerned with during that time, and a parenting game plan. Just as relevant are adolescent social-emotional changes, so we'll examine cultural norms and expectations of masculinity, gender identity, and expression. Consider all of this with an eye toward nurturing the overall well-being of a maturing teen, as they navigate inevitable pressures, feelings, and emotions, both intrinsically and extrinsically.

CHAPTER ONE

A Puberty Primer

Every journey has a starting point. In this chapter we'll start our voyage of discovery by focusing on the basics: what boys go through during puberty. This includes physical development, such as height and weight increases; overall body changes; and changes to the genitals. We'll also review physiological processes, including erections and ejaculation, and discuss why privacy is important to your son at this point in his life.

Going Through Puberty

Puberty changes for boys canin as early as age 9 and as late as age 14. The major changes that come with puberty generally take five to seven years. However, sometimes growth can continue for a decade of life. So physical growth that starts in puberty might be complete by age 16 or last as late as the early 20s. That's a wide-ranging start and end time, but it's because each person is on their own timeline.

One misconception about puberty growth is that people with testicles release testosterone, people with ovaries release estrogen, and that's it. But although testosterone is responsible for what are often deemed masculine characteristics, it's just one major hormone at play during puberty. All humans release testosterone, estrogen, and many more hormones; it's just a matter of when and how much. The various chemicals in the body that direct growth and development during puberty reach a balance that is unique to each individual.

Besides an increase in genital size, the typical first changes that a person with testicles will experience include the appearance of secondary sex characteristics like body hair, muscle growth, and a deepened voice. During adolescence, most boys will experience the biggest changes in the middle of their puberty timeline. Two to three years of consecutive growth spurts and physical maturity is typical, though as we've said, your mileage may vary.

Height and Weight

Physical size may not truly be the first sign of puberty in your son, but it is certainly one you'll notice early on. This is the one that relatives like to point out when visiting, and it's a metric that doctors and caretakers have been tracking since birth.

Fair warning, though: A teen or preteen boy may not be as open or excited about this as you are, especially in relation to their peers. Pointing out his weight gain—or lack thereof—can be taken the wrong way. Discussing their height may feel like a putdown instead of a fun jab.

It should go without stating that boys and men all have various body shapes . . . body positivity, remember? We may be bombarded with messages in the media of what constitutes a male physique, but make sure to instill the notion that boys can be healthy at any size.

GROWTH SPURTS

As you may have already witnessed, children often get heavier before getting taller. Shoulders can lag behind the hips, or feet can grow before the legs get longer. Even your son's head can seem different in proportion to the rest of his body. Puberty tends to bring on the fastest physical changes in a growing body since infancy. That's a tall order, but growth spurts play a big role, and they're not always synchronized.

For the most part, expect to see a growth spurt with your son getting quite a bit taller and/or heavier in just a year. This will happen several times between ages 9 and 18 or so. Also expect things to slow down from time to time, too. You might see a big difference between one annual doctor's visit and the next, but then not much change for a while. Both scenarios are normal and healthy.

It's important to remind your son that everyone is different, and comparisons about puberty milestones can be unfair. In some boys, the changes are very slight and take years to occur. Your child's pediatrician will know what to do if there are any health concerns; likewise, inquire with a specialist if you have questions about delayed onset or early puberty.

GROWING PAINS

It's not just a figure of speech. With a high rate of growth, boys sometimes develop soreness in their body, particularly the thighs (quadriceps), lower legs (calves), and in the back of the knees. The soreness can come and go throughout adolescence as muscle growth falls behind and catches up with bone growth. Although annoying, growing pains are usually not a concern, as long as they aren't concentrated in the joints. Check with your doctor if that's the case.

If your son is athletic, he may be at risk for repetitive injury issues like tendinitis or Osgood-Schlatter disease, both characterized by pain in, around, or below the kneecap. Pediatricians often do spine checks on a growing teen to determine that the vertebrae are aligned correctly. If there's an *S*- or *C*-shaped curvature present during a scoliosis diagnosis, take comfort in knowing there are treatments to correct this.

Some boys will notice swelling in and around their nipples as they hit puberty, particularly in mid-teen years. This is normal and can last between six months and two years. The term for this is *gynecomastia*. It means the tissue behind the nipples becomes enlarged and may even cause the nipples to become more sensitive during this time. Gynecomastia is rarely a concern, and swelling usually goes away on its own as the body balances hormone levels. If this is not the case, check with your family doctor.

Body Hair and Odor

Like most of the changes we explore, body hair will vary from person to person, boy to boy. It will all depend on genetics and hormones. No matter what gender or race, however, we all tend to have at least some arm and leg hair early in life. As puberty begins, boys generally see changes in body hair thanks to testosterone. The fine hair from childhood will become thicker and a bit longer.

In most boys, underarm, facial, and pubic hair will develop by age 16 and fill in for a few years before it arrives at adult length. The torso, including the chest and abdomen, can gain a little to a lot of hair by the end of puberty. This also tends to start by age 16, but much of it won't arrive until the end of adolescence or even into a man's 20s. Once again, genetics and testosterone are the major factors.

Puberty causes the sweat glands to become more active, and when sweat comes into contact with bacteria on the skin, the result can be body odor. If finances and access allow, families might opt for regular showers or baths, clean clothes, and deodorant. But it may take time and gentle encouragement for your son to develop these new habits.

KEEPING THINGS CLEAN

Upon the onset of puberty, it's smart for your son to start upping the attention he puts to overall hygiene. By ages 11 to 12, it's time for him to spend a bit more time washing his face, and as mentioned, deodorant should become part of his daily routine. With the genitals, it's important to care for the penis and testicles at any age, but upon puberty it will require even more of a focus since things are growing and becoming more sensitive. Whether intact or circumcised, boys should gently clean around the glans and foreskin of the penis while remaining careful not to put soap inside the urethra.

Make it a priority to help your son establish great hygiene habits. The earlier such routines are started, the easier it is to inquire about them as he progresses through puberty. If he gets neglectful about his hygiene, a straightforward comment is fine— you're the caregiver after all, so just say outright that he could use a shower or has been wearing that T-shirt for too many days without cleaning it.

Voice

A boy's Adam's apple will grow during puberty because the larynx—the voice box that controls the opening to the windpipe— is getting larger. The growing vocal cords and other tissues cause a deeper tone to the voice. Voice cracks are common by ages 12 to 13; the voice will change through age 16 or so, when it will settle in as a grown-up voice for the remainder of life. Until then, let your son know he can expect vocal highs and lows and a few squeaks in between. Encourage him to handle vocal cracks by either:

- ignoring them completely.
- giving a simple apology and moving on.
- maintaining a sense of humor about them.

Skin

As many as 85 percent of boys get acne during adolescence, because of the effect of hormones on the skin's oil glands. So your son won't be the only one to experience a pimple among his peers. Acne will be most common in the mid to late teen years, from age 13 onward.

Let your son know that most people get some acne during adolescence. It is caused by hormone changes; it doesn't mean the skin is dirty in any way. Someone with pimples might believe that lots of people are focused on their acne, but the reality is the opposite; most people don't notice it.

With this and other skin conditions like athlete's foot, plantar warts, eczema, psoriasis, or dermatitis, help your son monitor his hygiene, use simple over-the-counter creams, and/or consult a doctor or skin expert with questions.

Genitals

The testicles will generally grow first, before other genital changes kick in. The testes will gain size as well as sensitivity by ages 10 to 12. This will be gradual and mostly unnoticed. By ages 13 to 14, boys will then experience significant changes from childhood. The penis will grow in size and length as well, following the testicles from ages 10 to 14. It's typical for the genitals to also become a bit darker in skin color during puberty.

One of the more common questions from teenage boys is, "Is my penis normal?" If you get cornered on this topic, work to calm their mind. Penis length varies as much as the rest of human bodies. An adult flaccid penis is generally a few inches in length, and an erect penis potentially doubles that size. Measurements depend on genetics and individual anatomy. Everything is still growing during puberty and, just like height and weight, boys can be healthy at any size. There's no accurate research to suggest that diet, medication, exercise regime, or any factor besides surgery affects the size or shape of genitals.

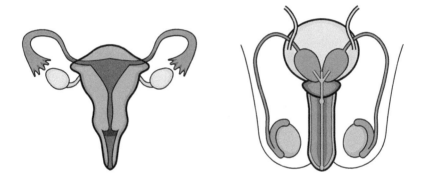

Erections

An erection happens when the spongy tissue inside the penis fills with blood and the organ becomes rigid, standing up and out from the body. Erections are normal and healthy. They will occur more often during puberty because hormones are helping the body grow and develop. During this time, erections can occur for seemingly no reason at all. Help your son know that when this happens, it's polite and private to keep that news to himself. For the most part, spontaneous erections go away in a matter of minutes. Boys will find more control over erections as they gain experience with age.

As with all anatomical changes, there are a few health issues to keep in mind. If you suspect any of these or notice other issues, be sure to check with your child's pediatrician.

Hydrocele: a type of swelling that occurs when fluid collects in the thin sheath surrounding a testicle. It is more common in young boys, but can still occur in teens and older men.

Peyronie's disease: a chronic condition that involves the development of abnormal scar tissue inside the penis, often resulting in bent or painful erections. It usually develops after the age of 18.

Phimosis: a condition in which the foreskin of an uncircumcised penis can't be retracted from the penis head, causing painful urination and erections. About 10 percent of boys are born with this condition.

Testicular torsion: when a testicle rotates, twisting the spermatic cord that brings blood to the scrotum. The reduced blood flow causes sudden and often severe pain and swelling. It's most common between ages 12 and 18, but it can occur at any age, even before birth.

Ejaculation

At the onset of puberty, sperm cells begin production in the testicles. This also means boys will develop the ability to ejaculate, or release sperm cells in semen. Semen is a white, clear-ish fluid that keeps sperm cells alive on their way out of the body. During wet dreams, masturbation, or sexual contact, semen can be released in waves of contracting pulses.

Anywhere between 50 million and 1 billion sperm can be released by a healthy adult man during this time. Amazingly, these cells are so small that they all fit into a single teaspoon of fluid. Ejaculation for men will most commonly coincide with pleasurable feelings of an orgasm. As the reproductive system starts to mature, ejaculation during sleep—aka nocturnal emissions or wet dreams—is not unusual. More on that topic to come.

The Importance of Privacy

The changes during puberty often cause young people to want more privacy in the bathroom and in the bedroom. This is normal; growing boys will understandably want to shower and change clothes behind closed doors. Privacy also makes it easier for them to handle sexual health matters like nocturnal emissions (wet dreams) and masturbation.

Privacy is an excellent precursor to sexual consent. Consent is the agreement between people for something to happen. Establishing and maintaining personal privacy is great way to practice respect and model consent—it reinforces the idea that nothing happens to our bodies and boundaries without communication. Honoring your son's privacy allows him to feel comfortable to open up to you when the time comes. He knows he has your respect. How you set up your lines of communication is up to the two of you, but certainly consider your son's privacy as a main issue to honor during his adolescence.

Avoid invading your son's privacy unless there are warning signs for concern:

- You overhear troubling news he shared with friends.
- Your son's grades have been abnormal.
- He's been quickly withdrawing from previous interests.
- He's getting in more trouble or showing an increase in disrespect.
- Your son has been hiding things from you.

Masturbation

If the topic of erections or masturbation comes up, it can catch parents slightly off guard. But boys know early on that erections happen, so a matter-of-fact answer is probably all that is warranted. If the word "erection" feels too clinical, saying "when hard" is a perfectly acceptable alternative.

It's important to remain body-positive and avoid shame during these discussions. You may have values around this subject that you want to plug during such a conversation, but ensure you are doing so with the truth: From a physiological and scientific perspective, masturbation is not an unhealthy act. There is certainly a time and place for self-touch, but it is generally a positive and safe way for people to explore their sexuality and know their own bodies. Even daily self-pleasure is not cause for alarm. There are caveats to this. Consider intervening if:

▸ Self-pleasure is taking away from social time with friends or family.
▸ Masturbation has become physically painful.
▸ Self-touch and/or pornography use has become compulsive or has altered real-life interactions (misogynistic comments, inappropriate mention or description, etc.).

Should a course correction be needed, here are some ways to help:

▸ Respect privacy, and remain body-positive in all discussions.
▸ Impart that self-touch is done in private and at appropriate times.
▸ Have separate body lotion or lube available for his personal use.
▸ Refrain from interruption or humiliation.

Seek counseling if masturbation or porn use seems to be out of control. A full chapter on navigating pornography can be found in part III of this book.

Wet Dreams

Erections will happen overnight throughout puberty and into adulthood. This is part of the body's sleep cycle. Blood flow increases and decreases during sleep, and at some point the body might release semen out of the penis. This is called a *nocturnal emission*, or wet dream; it's a bodily reaction to the increase of the hormone testosterone. Wet dreams are healthy and normal. Some boys might have wet dreams every week or two, others might not have them more than a few times throughout puberty.

For privacy purposes, this might be a good time to teach your son to do his own laundry, if you have the means. He'll appreciate the ability to discreetly clean his own clothing in case of wet dreams. Like everything with sexual wellness, avoid shame at all costs.

KEEP IN MIND

- Puberty changes for boys will begin as early as age 9 and as late as age 14. Puberty generally takes five to seven years, but everyone's body is on its own timeline.
- New hygiene habits for adolescent boys should include skin care, regular showers, deodorant use, and extra attention to the penis and testicles.
- The developing body gets things ready and functioning correctly during puberty in preparation for adulthood. Part of that process includes an increase in erections, a potential for wet dreams, and even masturbation. All of these are normal and healthy and might require more privacy for your child.
- Personal privacy is not only a practical concern, but it is also a great way to practice respect and model consent. It reinforces the notion that nothing happens to our bodies and boundaries without communication.

CHAPTER TWO

What It Means to Be a "Man"

Social and emotional development for boys have always been shaped by cultural norms. Many of the gender roles of previous centuries, even from the childhoods of adults living today, don't hold true any longer. It's no longer assumed that men work to provide for their families by earning a wage for food and shelter while women take care of domestic issues, caring for children and running the home. In this chapter we will discuss what it means to become a man in modern times. We'll examine the evolving definition of masculinity and the traits surrounding this term, as well as the social and emotional lives of boys. All of these factors affect your son's experience during puberty, and they may be quite different from what you yourself experienced at his age.

From Boys to Men

Currently, adolescent boys grow up in a culture with gender roles in flux. Much of the world is fighting the notion that mothers nurture and fathers protect; that boys should learn to fight and girls should learn to cook. All of these roles and behaviors have worth, but anyone can see that the stereotyped gender expectations are detrimental to individuals and society.

Without a doubt, the first thing that stands out when considering such stereotypes is that a woman's role in society is deserving of so much more. And because of this, a man's role in society is also reinventing itself. Arguably, then, striving for gender equity includes a revamped role of what it means to be a man. This can cause a conflict of emotions in growing boys.

Trying to reconcile the necessary push to dismantle domestic and workplace inequities toward women along with powerful gender expectations to be a strong male presence, it's easy to see why boys might not know where they should stand. On a larger societal scale, this challenge is to keep the positive aspects of masculinity while updating or eliminating those that are outdated and harmful. Closer to home for parents, the question becomes: How can we help our sons develop socially and emotionally so they can form healthy adult relationships?

Let's take a closer look at some of the missteps that you can help your son avoid as he finds his footing and chooses his path.

Egocentrism

It may sometimes seem as though your son is as self-centered as a toddler, but that's a natural part of development through adolescence. Boys in this age group do have the capability to develop compassion and empathy, but only through a personal lens. This is true for everyone in adolescence, in fact, not just people who identify as male as they are growing.

Because social-emotional competence takes years to develop, boys are often called emotionally immature. Rightfully so, and sometimes true enough for parents to shake their heads in frustration. But let's think of this as a truth instead of an insult.

Parents can help with their child's worldview development by consistently finding learning opportunities in current events, from history, or by sharing relevant stories from their own youth. Even an older teenage boy can be in need of examples and reminders to step out of the spotlight and take a proverbial walk in someone else's shoes. This is important work for healthy future relationships and sexual contact. A general compassion for others will have a direct impact on their capacity to care about, listen to, collaborate with, and deeply connect with a partner.

Defining "Toxic Masculinity"

Being male in itself is not toxic. Growing up, a boy deserves just as much celebration as a girl or nonbinary individual. There is no shame in having masculinity, in expressing masculine characteristics, or in being a proud, respectful young man. Toxic masculinity, on the other hand, is indeed harmful. It purports the extreme notion that manliness is only intertwined with power, domination, violence, and sexism.

In sports, this toxic attitude can manifest itself when an athlete pushes to play through injury. In music, movies, art, and video games, toxic masculinity favors aggression and violence to a fault; opting to avoid anything deemed too feminine because being in touch with a more sensitive side means you forfeit your "man card." In same-sex friendships, toxic masculinity can show up as homophobia, and in dating relationships, it can be expressed as emotional disconnection. In sexual relationships, toxic masculinity can manifest as persuasion for conquest.

According to research by the World Health Organization and related studies, the more men conform to toxic norms, the more likely they are to engage in risky behaviors, including excessive alcohol and tobacco use, reckless driving, and skipping needed sleep. In addition, these men are more likely to view such risky choices as normal. Toxic masculinity creates stigma for mental health treatment, fueling the perception that depression, anxiety, and related social-emotional issues are weaknesses and that seeking counseling or therapy is unmanly.

Toxic masculinity stands in striking contrast to being a gentleman, a term often used for positive masculine behavior: providing safety; supporting fair play and competition; creating/building/repairing; and striving for success. Being a gentleman—or whatever term you prefer for it—is a great way to harness the positive characteristics of masculinity by aspiring to embody polite, chivalrous thoughts and behavior. A gentleman is kind, respectful, helpful, and courteous—traits we welcome as caregivers and want to help our sons develop.

A MACHO MENTALITY

There are times to be tough and, equally, there are times to be emotionally vulnerable. Vulnerability, in the positive context, means acknowledging difficult emotions instead of avoiding or repressing them. Being macho—always acting strong, never admitting to weakness—might not be what you or your son would consider being a gentleman. Toxic, macho statements can appear under the guise of grit and tenacity: "I don't need to ask for directions, I know where I'm going." "I don't need a physical check-up—never been stronger."

We can help our sons by showing them how a macho mentality ignores a holistic sense of maleness to focus only on bravado, becoming a parody of masculinity itself. Phrases like "be a man" or "man up" are typically harmful. More helpful phrasing might be, "Sorry to hear you made a bad decision. It could be time to admit to your mistake and apologize—wouldn't you agree? Explain how you were wrong in this instance and go from there."

BOYS WILL BE BOYS

The message behind the problematic expression "boys will be boys" is that there are some inherent tendencies of people growing up male. That may be true to some degree, but the phrase is often used to excuse invasive competitiveness or aggression, as if harming others is allowed because boys are just fulfilling gender norms. Sure, wrestling and physical play is a part of growing up, and boys can certainly roughhouse as part of their development. But we shouldn't condone it when our sons make unsafe decisions to impress their peers. We shouldn't allow degradation of girls, women, queer folks, gender-nonconforming people, or any other group of people that is marginalized because of how they identify. As parents, our word choices always matter. Avoiding this kind of apologist phrasing will help with personal accountability for young men everywhere.

INGRAINED MISOGYNY

Ultimately, the most extreme side effect of toxic masculinity is prejudice and violence toward others, especially those who identify as female. This exhibits itself through all sorts of speech and actions that favor men over women. Centuries of patriarchal culture, the tendency for men to average higher in physical size and strength, and the depiction of gender roles in media and advertising have perpetuated these notions. These factors work in combination with ongoing cultural norms that assert that men should bond with other men and hold allegiance to gender above other relationships—the offensive "bros before hoes" mentality of recent decades. Bringing the ugly nature of misogyny to light for our sons, including the legacy of historical misogynistic discrimination, can help them be on guard that their concept of masculinity doesn't morph from healthy and positive to toxic and violent.

Sexual Prowess

In regard to sexual wellness, toxic masculinity concepts can be intrinsically harmful for your son, sparking unrealistic expectations of a boy's sexual appetite: "I'm a guy, does that mean I should want sex more?" Toxic masculinity can bring performance anxiety ("I've heard I should be able to last hours and hours during sex . . . what's wrong with me?"). It can affect and harm other people, too. Toxic masculinity can lead to prioritizing one's personal pleasure above relationship connections ("I just really need to get laid tonight."). And it can be used to justify assault and other misconduct ("Is this a game where I'm supposed to keep trying and trying until they give in?").

However, remember the principle of sex positivity. It's important to convey to your son that simply having sexual urges and interests is not toxic and doesn't equate to sexual misconduct or deviance.

The Social Life of Boys

Societal norms and expectations placed on men impact a boy's thoughts and behavior, but your son will still grow up with a unique personality with plenty to contribute to social relationships. Just because you are preparing to help him through turbulent times doesn't mean he won't have a great adolescence. Case in point: his social life.

Often, media stereotypes can give people the wrong idea about teenage life. Teens don't argue with siblings every day, and they don't rebel against their parents each weekend. It's important to realize what is normal, what you can expect, and what can help your son remain socially healthy as he ages.

Interests change. You can expect adolescents to lose interest in some aspects of their childhood, even hobbies and activities they seemed obsessed with. This is absolutely normal and even to be encouraged. We want our children to adapt and update interests as they age to make way for newfound enjoyment in clubs, teams, or after-school events.

Extracurricular activities loom large. In fact, they'll get just as much focus as academics, if not more. This is important because your son is branching out to make new friends and build relationships beyond the classroom, which are often deeper than the ones formed throughout the school day.

His schedule becomes busy. Your son may also find ways to participate in community events, including summer camps and art, music, and technology clubs. He might surprise you by liking or being good at an activity he never tried before. Keep the doors of opportunity open for him as much as access and finances allow—and as much as he'll let you.

Shifting Relationship Priorities

Adolescence will bring a shift in your son's social agenda. Teens tend to move from focusing on family to focusing on friends and then, potentially, focusing on dating relationships. School and other activities will revolve around classmates. That doesn't mean your son will neglect family. In fact, he will want things running smoothly at home so he has a constant, safe environment to return to each day. Boys can act differently in front of close family compared to peers, venting at home after keeping it together throughout the day. A lot of this is because your son has an established trust that his parents and siblings will be there for him, no matter what.

To do your part, keep communication lines open with constant questions, even if he offers one-word answers. He might seem annoyed, but at least he knows you care. And that can make the difference when he needs answers about sexual health or other delicate matters. You can coax a bit more conversation by avoiding questions that can be answered in a word or two. Instead of "How was your day?" try, "What's one thing you are proud of today?" or "What's been good lately?" It's harder for him to be curt with those kinds of prompts, plus they help him focus on positives.

Following the Crowd

Your son may follow friends or crush interests into places and pursuits that he doesn't actually like that much. He might "try on" personalities for a while, attempting to impress his buddies—or that certain someone. You may have to allow him to find out for himself the best way to create and maintain his place on the social ladder. Be on standby, though, if you notice a preoccupation with popularity and need to intervene with gentle observations. If he denies you any involvement, let it be; he'll need to come to a conclusion himself. Should it turn out he made a wrong move, remain supportive without any scolding. No one ever feels better after hearing "I told you so."

Caveat: In the event that your son follows peer pressure into illegal or unsafe activities, absolutely do get involved. As a caregiver this is your chance to relay your values and have a direct discussion about specific activities. Be sure to separate the behavior from the child, though. He's not necessarily a bad kid because he did something wrong, even on repeated occasions. To eliminate unseemly habits, try to be open about the reasoning. Adolescent boys want to know the *why* behind any edicts or punishments. This will take conversation—not a compromise, but a debate that you may not particularly want. Nevertheless, it sets a good precedent for resolving issues related to relationship health and sexual wellness.

THE OUTSIZE IMPORTANCE OF SAME-SEX FRIENDSHIPS

As adolescents shift their social focus from family to friendships, their peers can become like a second family. Many boys find their closest bonds in same-sex friendships, full of camaraderie and kinship.

Boys who spend time together find empathy and solidarity in shared life experiences; they talk through their worries and advise each other. This is normal and worthy of its own celebration. Same-sex friendships can in fact provide positive companionship and guidance.

However, it's a good idea to keep an eye on your son's circle of friends, to the degree you're able. You can't choose his friends for him, but a discussion is warranted if you notice any of these signs of potential toxic masculinity:

- Demeaning, misogynistic, homophobic, transphobic, and racist comments by your son, and if his friends encourage them.
- Prioritization of his same-sex friendships to an unhealthy degree, creating a closed-minded attitude and "othering" of different genders.
- Fear that he'll be ostracized if he doesn't behave in an offensive or insulting manner toward those outside the group.

Head off unhealthy friendships by modeling healthy behavior, letting your son see the importance of various types of friendships in your own life. Reinforce positivity in regard to your son's treatment of various interests, priorities, and lifestyles: "Hey, I think it's great that you hang out with so many different kinds of kids, and I'm proud that you remain open to meeting new people of various backgrounds."

Comparison to Peers

In certain circumstances, comparison can bring out a healthy competitiveness—academics, sports, musical or dramatic performance—but for the most part, it deflates our self-esteem instead. Comparison can get particularly tricky for parenting through subjects of puberty and sex because boys are on their own timelines, plus a young person's sexuality is such a personal topic. Just as teens can brag and exaggerate, so can parents—as strange as that sounds.

Comparing notes with a trusted friend who's also raising a teen can help you share angles on bridging tough topics and evaluate what works versus what doesn't. Just keep in mind that you're not in competition, and that differences in values and personality styles can limit how effective one parent's practices will work for another.

Teens and preteens will also need reminders that comparing themselves to their peers is of limited value, especially when it comes to the wildly varying time frames that puberty milestones can follow. Growth spurts, body hair, and other physical changes will happen in their own time, and there's no benefit to treating puberty like a competition.

When it comes to sports, academics, and other activities—some of which are explicitly competitive—comparisons with peers will occur, and that's natural. But watch for excessive comparison, which can stop your son from trying. Work to reinforce a growth mindset, focusing on effort over output. Praise the process. This sounds like:

"You didn't win. But did you do your absolute best? Can you change anything for next time?"

"Looks like you spent a lot of time on that project! The attention to detail must have been difficult but fun."

"I like how you are working toward that music piece—you missed some notes, huh? Are you going to keep practicing?"

Use the power of "yet" if your son brings up his friends or classmates while criticizing himself. "You're right. You can't do that . . . yet." This simple statement affirms your son's position and feelings, conveys your affirmation, and offers a growth mindset wrapped up in a few words.

The Emotional Life of Boys

If the teenage boy in your home is the size of the other adults, you may start treating him as equally mature. It's important to note that their physical development is in no way parallel to their emotional development. The teenage brain experiences feelings the same way that an adult brain does. But the rational, decision-making part of their brain is not quite there yet. In fact, those brain circuits won't fully develop until the early 20s and will continue to mature throughout life.

This means that your teenage son may not handle his emotions well. It's not a choice; he's simply not wired that way. The disappointment of a canceled event, the anger of a failing friendship, the loneliness of not being invited out—these can all be met with an intense "end-of-the-world" reaction. Something quite inconsequential, such as missing schoolwork or, yes, even spilled milk, can be blown out of proportion. Be prepared to emphasize that whatever the issue, everything isn't ruined. When the meltdown's over, offer nonjudgmental suggestions on how to respond appropriately to a setback, and allow him the time he needs to practice and grow that life skill.

Your son's ability to regulate his emotions can improve his communication with others and, in turn, achieve true intimacy with a partner. Pleasurable sexual relationships will require as much, if not more, of an emotional connection as a physical connection.

Mood Swings

Emotions have a place in life. We don't want negative thoughts to stick around, naturally, but many of our least favorite feelings give us important insight into current circumstances. For example, what is frustration telling us? How come deep feelings of disappointment are showing up? Is this really anger, or is it covering up hurt and sadness? Leaning in to learn one's personal tendencies is empowering, so encourage your son to be curious about the causes and sources of his moods and emotions.

Your son's emotional ups and downs will be as unique as any physical trait. Some boys have weekly roller coasters during puberty, whereas others stay on a relatively even keel month to month. This can change depending on age and development stage. Early on, the mood swings might be slight, then increase in intensity for a few years before calming down again by ages 18 to 19.

Whatever the case, parents can help by doing their best not to dismiss their son's emotions as juvenile. It may seem like your son's high points are "manic" and his lows are "depressive," but be careful of labeling them as such, since that trivializes real emotional disorders. If there is ever concern, let your son's doctor know so you can get a referral to a mental health expert. Otherwise, expect ebbs and flows. Not everything needs a parental lesson; sometimes just sitting with him to share an emotion like disappointment is enough to show care and affirmation.

Emotional Suppression

Repeatedly throwing around demands to "grow up" or "suck it up" at a teen or preteen boy can prove emotionally devastating. In a developing brain, enforcing toughness as a virtue above all other emotional responses in life means feelings such as sadness, frustration, and disappointment are pushed aside, and the complexities of emotions like compassion, gratitude, and love don't have a place to develop. Those emotions continue to exist, but with no way to express them for fear of ridicule or shame, they can instead manifest as anger. Sometimes humor will be used by teen boys as a coping mechanism, often inappropriately if they're discouraged from expressing a full spectrum of emotions. Parents can help their sons find healthy avenues for emotional expression by modeling such behavior themselves; finding examples in books, music, movies, and games; and being available to talk through the root problems after a tantrum or outburst has passed.

Anger and Aggression

Even if you don't discourage your child from expressing his emotions, toxic masculinity and other societal pressures may inhibit him from doing so. So it could be that anger tends to be the first emotion to surface in your adolescent son—or at least the first to show itself to others in any given situation. Be ready at all times to help him see the root of the angst. Ask questions—not to pry, but to help him learn and cope: "What are you mad about?" "Why is that so annoying to you?" Unless it's immediately dangerous to do so, allow the anger to exist by confirming how frustrated and hurt your son must feel.

Consider yourself when angry—do you want someone in your face telling you to calm down? It doesn't help, right? Same for your son. Work with him to find appropriate ways of experiencing stress, without throwing or breaking things. Then gently push to discover the cause and find out if the issue can be addressed. Ensure he takes the lead in weighing possible solutions; don't try to fix things for him. Use descriptive words to correctly model how he's feeling, even if it's being expressed as anger: Is he sad, deceived, heartbroken, guilty, unprepared, stressed, tired, overwhelmed?

Aggression is different from anger. An increased tendency toward aggression can be a natural result of increased testosterone levels, or it could be a consequence of particular events and environments. When harnessed correctly as competitiveness, it can help boys in their hobbies and interests. As anyone with athletic experience knows, competitive edge is gained by using the energy of aggression to push the threshold of one's physical and mental capabilities. Competitiveness in other endeavors like art, music, and technology can also lead to breakthroughs. The trick is to help your son understand when and how to use aggressive behavior for positive purposes. Rather than trying to diminish competitive tendencies, work on finding an appropriate time and place for expressing them—competitive behavior while playing a baseball game makes sense; on a dinner date, it does not. Revisit a specific instance where he was overwhelming with his aggression to spotlight other possibilities. Avoid an accusatory tone in order to teach instead of reprimand.

AN EPIDEMIC OF MALE LONELINESS

We're in the midst of an epidemic of loneliness for adult men. Surveys have found that as many as 44 percent of males age 18 and older say they feel lonely all the time. Men are 50 percent more likely than women to say they don't have any close friends and 33 percent more likely to say they don't have a best friend.

It's more than an issue of mood or psychology; loneliness can be a matter of life and death. Experts point to loneliness as a direct cause of addiction; men have significantly higher rates of smoking, drinking, and using substances than women. The same is evident with increasing rates of suicide—male loneliness has been called a "ticking time bomb" causing men to disproportionately take their own lives. Research tells us that men die by suicide 3.6 times more often than women. In addition, psychologists suggest a two-way relationship with male loneliness and excessive internet pornography use, each feeding the other.

As a generalization, adult men can grow apart from adolescent friends because they lack the communication skills to maintain avenues of contact. A phone call, email, or text message goes unsent because of learned helplessness, for fear of being snubbed, or because of gender norms.

Your son does not have to grow into this fate. Take action by teaching him that it's healthy and normal for men to keep up with friends, that boys can have friends of a different gender, and that communication skills transfer to crushes, dating, and love interests. Does he know it's okay to talk about feelings or share personal thoughts about a book, movie, or art project?

Don't let a narrow understanding of friendship condemn your son to a lonely future.

Shame and Embarrassment

Shame is a tricky emotion. Although it can keep us conscious of wrongdoing or immoral behavior, feeling shamed by others is humiliation. It leads to distress or mental anguish. Embarrassment is a more useful emotion. It's a feeling we impose on ourselves—one that's less stigmatizing than shame, but provides enough mental discomfort to act as a life lesson. Repeated or excessive embarrassment can be harmful, but in general, embarrassment is instructional. Shame is traumatic.

What this means is that parents of boys growing through adolescence should give them room to feel embarrassed but avoid inflicting shame. Take for example the embarrassment after burping too loudly in public. This can create social awkwardness, with feelings of guilt connected to the action itself. But taking your son to task for such an occurrence, and making him feel he's inadequate because of it, puts the guilt on him, not the behavior, and can lead to social anxiety.

Applied to sexual health, embarrassment about nudity in a locker room is normal. But feeling shame for exploring one's own body through masturbation is detrimental. The damage that shame can do to a boy is another reason that caregivers will want to remain body- and sex-positive. Stay far away from shaming your son over any natural physical growth or curiosity about sexual topics.

Adolescents of all genders can develop nervousness about locker rooms, public restrooms, or changing rooms. Assure your son he's not the first to have that concern, if it shows up. This quick and truthful statement may work to help him overcome embarrassment: "Everyone in there is more focused on doing their own thing than noticing you."

KEEP IN MIND

- Positive masculinity can include, but is not limited to: respect, courtesy, fair competition, creating/building/ repairing, and striving for success—and, most important, consent.
- Toxic masculinity is the extreme notion that manliness is only intertwined with power, domination, violence, and sexism.
- The social life of boys can include shifting relationships, situational personality changes, a crowd mentality, and comparisons to peers.
- The teenage brain isn't equipped for full emotional management. But learning to regulate their growing emotional well-being can help teen boys handle mood swings and move from emotional suppression to emotional expression.
- Parents can help their son by reinforcing ideas of positive masculinity and by drawing attention to the complex emotions that may be underlying their son's anger or aggression.

CHAPTER THREE

Gender, Sex, and Sexual Health

Today, more than ever, sex education requires more than explaining the fundamentals of sex. It's really about preparing and supporting your son as he grows and develops. Sexual health and wellness have a huge impact on who he is, what he stands for, how he sees the world, and how he treats others. In this chapter, we touch on those concepts so you can help your son sort through life experiences that will exert an ever-lasting influence on how he approaches gender, sex, and his sexual wellness.

A Strong Sense of Self

Fielding difficult questions and explaining complicated issues around sexuality are important tasks for the parents of an adolescent boy. But one of the most significant influences a parent can contribute to their son's sexual health is to give him a strong sense of self. That doesn't mean feeding his ego with accolades. Your real job as a parent is to truly understand your child's strengths and weakness and help him navigate those waters with grace, ease, and resiliency. Cultivating the following three qualities in your son will enable his sense of self to flourish:

Self-Awareness. Support your son in developing a positive self-concept so he can observe and evaluate his own thoughts and actions without shame. Encourage him to remind himself that no one is perfect, we cannot be perfectly defined by labels, and even our own thoughts can sabotage our ability to be content.

Self-Affirmation. Even just a few truths relevant to your son's personal style can break down negative self-images and build up positive vibes. For example, if your son is insecure about his physique, suggest that he focus on function versus form: "I am pretty good at _____. It's challenging but fun." Remind him to concentrate on what he can do instead of what he can't do: "I can get better at _____ today." Make him mindful of the differences he can make: "I have a good sense of humor. I'm also creative with _____."

Self-Care. Teenagers may feel indestructible, but they still need to attend to their health. Doing so not only boosts overall well-being, but also builds a sense of self through habits of valuing, and being responsible for, one's physical wellness. To that end, encourage your son to include a variety of healthy activity types in his schedule:

- **Focus time** to set goals and challenges.
- **Creative time** for spontaneous and creative activities.

- ▸ **Social time** for relaxing and interacting with friends and others.
- ▸ **Active time** for exercise and movement that strengthens the mind and body.
- ▸ **Down time** to relax and decompress with music, movies, games, and hobbies.
- ▸ **Inward time** for quiet reflection and setting future expectations.
- ▸ **Sleep time** to allow the body and brain to recover from the day and consolidate life experiences.

Gender Identity and Expression

Whatever path your child takes to become a fully realized adult, it's important that you both understand the distinction between sex and gender. Let's first examine the meaning behind these terms as well as some related vocabulary. Use this background to guide your own education, but mostly for affirmation of your son's identity and expression. Perhaps he's showing signs of questioning his own identity—trying out different looks in terms of clothing, hair, and accessories, for example—or interacting with friends or peers who are dealing with identity questions. In either case, these insights will help your child feel supported and will aid them in exploration and making positive decisions.

Sex

When referencing an individual's anatomy, sex is a biological concept based on appearance of genitalia and other reproductive organs. Sex can also be classified based on chromosomes and hormone levels.

Gender

In contrast to anatomical sex, gender is a social construct that describes characteristics such as behavior, social and relationship roles, and how those attributes are expressed. Gender involves an individual's perceptions of themselves, as well as society's interaction with that perception. Think of sex and gender in this context: Sex is mostly physical, whereas gender is mainly mental, emotional, and social.

Gender Identity

Gender identity is best described as the way a person feels in regard to their own gender and how self-concept and gender roles impact each other. Gender identity can begin before puberty. However, for most kids, it forms throughout adolescence and well into adulthood. Gender can be identified as male, female, nonbinary, gender neutral, transgender, agender, pangender, genderqueer, or all, none, or a combination of these. Help your child understand that it's okay for them, or anyone, to not categorize their gender identity if that's how they want it. And also explain that gender identity can slide anywhere on that spectrum throughout life.

Gender Expression

Gender expression is what people present to the world regarding their gender identity. Gender expression is a choice of what we allow others to see, including but not limited to clothing, hairstyle, jewelry, makeup, and other accessories. Let your child know that however they choose to express their gender identity is up to them and that they should respect others' choices as well.

Gender Dysphoria

Gender dysphoria is the discomfort or distress that occurs in people who feel a mismatch between their assigned sex and their gender identity. Having a certain identity but expressing another can also cause a disconnect that might feed gender dysphoria.

Cisgender

Cisgender refers to a person whose gender identity is the same as their sex or gender assigned at birth. You may come across the shortened term *cis*; it means the same thing.

Transgender

Transgender is a term for anyone whose gender identity does not match their sex or gender assigned at birth. Estimates vary, but at the time of publishing, around 1 in 10,000 people are transgender. You may come across the shortened term *trans*; it means the same thing.

Making Sense of It All

There's been a lot of positive change in the media lately regarding gender identity. However, as a society we still have a way to go. For many children assigned male, they may not realize their gender identity until they begin going through puberty and experiencing changing secondary sexual characteristics. For many trans or gender-nonconforming people, puberty can be torture because physical changes and gender identity may not align. You may or may not see signs that your child is struggling, confused, or uncertain about their gender identity. As you navigate these moments, remember that gender identity is different for everyone.

One of the best practices is to have resources at the ready for any conversation your child wants to have. And most important, be sure that your child knows that you are there for them, no matter what. Let your child know that sex and gender are better considered as a continuum—meaning they are a fluid spectrum rather than two mutually exclusive categories of male and female. Although we may continue to see and hear the uproar of people fighting to maintain strict gender norms by claiming biology is binary, that is simply not the truth. Even chromosome patterns are not solely XX (considered female) and XY (considered male). XXY, XXYY, and other variations exist.

In other words, a binary classification system for sex or gender is inaccurate since there are more than two configurations, even if two of them are more common than others. As a caregiver, understanding this can help not only if your child falls into a nonbinary sex or gender category, but if family or friends do as well. Discussing this with your son is an instance of modeling awareness and celebrating gender diversity.

It's important to know that sex and gender roles vary from society to society, and our collective views of both can change over time. For example, sex and gender are generally assigned at birth and have historically been a binary designation of male or female, boy or girl. Recently, some parents are requesting that their child not be assigned a sex at birth. Some hospitals around the world are recording other designations, including nonbinary, indeterminate, intersex, and unknown, on birth certificates.

Pronouns

Pronoun usage is an important factor in validating someone's gender identity and normalizing the awareness, acceptance, and celebration of everyone's unique human characteristics. The English language is adopting more gender neutral singular pronouns, since a binary choice of "he" or "she" doesn't match everyone's gender identity. When someone's proper name isn't being used, some common nonbinary (neopronoun) options include *ze* or *xe* (substitutes for he or she, both pronounced "zee"), and *zir* or *hir* (for him or her, rhyming with "here"). The most common non-gendered pronouns at the time of this writing are "they" in place of he/she and "them" for him/her. The singular use of "they/them" has been used for centuries; it is in fact grammatically correct if your child—or anyone in your child's life—would like to use these for themselves.

Understanding this use of language is helpful for your son to know that he has options in his identity and expression. It also helps him be open and accepting to his peers. When in doubt, one can ask, "What are your pronouns?" or use "they/them" until advised otherwise.

Discussions about pronouns are opportunities for you to relay the message to your son that questioning things related to gender and sexuality is allowed, and he doesn't have to know everything about himself by his teenage years. Expressing a non-male gender isn't "trying to get attention" or "going through a phase." Teens figure things out as they age, which means gender expression might change, but parents can remain supportive no matter what. You love your child unconditionally because of their personality, not because of their pronouns.

Developing Sexual Interest

Sexuality is the awareness, acceptance, and enjoyment of our own body and the bodies of others. This includes sexual orientation, that is, what stimulates attraction for us and who/what we desire in relationships. "Sexuality" is a better term for this than "sexual preference," since most aspects of attraction aren't really preferred; they simply *exist*. Sexuality can include romantic attraction, which considers deeper intellectual and emotional qualities, or it can simply be physical in nature. You can think of it this way: Our anatomy is our body parts, our identity is our innate notion of self or feelings, our expression is our appearance, and our sexuality includes the attractions we may have.

Your son's interest in sexuality will depend on quite a few things. Physical maturation matters, since testosterone and sperm cell production can bring on sexual thoughts and attractions. This can start as early as ages 9 to 10, or it may begin in the mid-teenage years around ages 15 to 16. Societal factors also play a part, meaning boys tend to become aware of sex earlier than they are interested in it. Peers or the media might fuel intrigue, and relationships with emotional bonds can stir an increasing sexual desire through adolescence. It is natural to feel uninterested in, or even repulsed by, sexuality early in puberty. It's also natural to have a healthy curiosity about sex as soon as one becomes aware of it.

Here are a few more terms relating to gender and/or sexual identity and expression. Use this list to equip yourself with proper terminology for conversations with your son, either related to his own sexuality or that of others. Although people aren't always accurately defined by labels—and labels can certainly change throughout life—sometimes they can help if a teen is searching for self-awareness.

Lesbian and Gay

The terms lesbian and gay depend on a person's identity, expression, and attraction. Gay is used interchangeably in same sex/gender relationships and is currently considered respectful. "Homosexual" is an outdated, offensive term as it and its variations are used in antigay speech.

Bisexual

Generally speaking, bisexual is a term used to describe someone who is attracted to both the same gender and other genders, though not necessarily equally or at the same time.

Queer

This describes a person whose gender identity and/or gender expression falls outside of the societal norm for their assigned sex. This is a term used as a catchall by many people who in the past may have described themselves as lesbian or gay. In recent years this term has been reclaimed by the LGBTQIA community and is not longer considered an offensive term.

Asexual

Asexual is a term to describe a person who is not attracted to any sex or gender. Asexuality is different from deciding not to have sexual contact with anyone (abstinence or celibacy).

Pansexual

A person who is pansexual is attracted to another person of any sex and/or gender. Many people who identify as pansexual say their attraction is usually focused on personality rather than gender.

Sex and Sexual Health

Whatever the gender identity and sexuality of your child, it's important to understand the terminology around sex and sexual health. A well-vetted vocabulary equips them with the ability to have an informed discussion about sex and to engage in safe, pleasurable sex if it occurs. In chapter two we talked about wet dreams and masturbation that are specific to male anatomy. In this section we are going to review a few more important and inclusive terms regarding sex and sexual health, so your conversations can be helpful and informative.

Abstinence: This when a person chooses to refrain from having sex of any kind, not just penile-vaginal sex. Abstinence can be for a specific amount of time or over a lifetime. This is the only behavior that is 100 percent effective at preventing pregnancy and sexually transmitted infections (STIs).

Virginity: This is a societal construct that puts a lot of pressure on people to refrain from having penile-vaginal sex. Virginity is a journey into being a sexual person with others. Virginity is not something to "lose" so much as it is intimacy to gain.

Oral sex: This involves sex contact that includes mouth to vulva, mouth to penis, or mouth to anus. Some young people may think that oral sex isn't technically "sex." That perception may vary from generation to generation, but one thing to instill is that oral sex is in fact a type of sexual intimacy. Unprotected oral sex can transmit STIs.

Vaginal sex: Some people may only think of penile-vaginal sex as the standard definition of sex here. However, vaginal sex can also involve inserting other objects into the vagina or vulva to vulva contact. Unprotected penile-vaginal sex can result in a pregnancy and/or transmission of an STI. Vulva to vulva sex can transmit STIs.

Anal sex: This refers to sexual behaviors that involve inserting a penis or other object into the anus. Unprotected anal sex can transmit STIs.

Sexually Transmitted Infections

Before your child begins to have sex, it's important that they know the risks. Here are a few terms to help navigate those inevitable conversations.

Chlamydia: This is the most commonly reported STI, according to the Centers for Disease Control and Prevention (CDC). It is caused by a bacteria. Symptoms include pain during sex or urination, green or yellow discharge from the penis or vagina, and/or pain in the lower abdomen. However, some people have no symptoms at all. If left untreated, chlamydia can cause infections of the urethra, prostate gland, or testicles; pelvic inflammatory disease; and infertility.

Gonorrhea: This is another common bacterial STI. Similar to chlamydia, gonorrhea may produce no symptoms. If there are symptoms, they can include a white, yellow, beige, or green-colored discharge from the penis or vagina; pain or discomfort during sex or urination; frequent urination; and a sore throat. Gonorrhea can cause infections of the urethra, prostate gland, or testicles; pelvic inflammatory disease; and infertility.

Syphilis: This is yet another bacterial infection that often goes unnoticed in its early stages. The first symptom is usually a small round sore, known as a chancre. It can develop on the genitals, anus, or mouth. The sore may be painless but is very infectious. Further symptoms can include fever, fatigue, rash, headaches, joint pain, and weight and hair loss. If left untreated, late-stage syphilis can lead to loss of hearing, vision, or memory; mental illness; heart disease; infection of the brain or spinal cord; and death.

Hepatitis B: This is a virus found in infected blood, semen, and vaginal fluid and can be transmitted through unprotected sex. It's also spread through contaminated needles and syringes. Symptoms include fever, fatigue, nausea, dark urine, and clay-colored bowel movements.

Herpes simplex virus (HSV): There are two main strains of this virus: HSV-1 and HSV-2. Both can be transmitted sexually. The CDC estimates more than 1 out of 6 people ages 14 to 49 in the United States have herpes. HSV-1 causes oral herpes, which is responsible for cold sores or blisters. However, it can also be passed from a person's mouth to another person's genitals during oral sex. HSV-2 primarily causes genital herpes sores to develop on or around the genitals.

Human papillomavirus (HPV): This virus is passed from one person to another through intimate skin-to-skin or sexual contact. There are many different strains of the virus. The most common symptom of HPV is warts on the genitals, mouth, or throat. Some strains can lead to cancer, including cancer of the mouth, cervix, or rectum.

Human immunodeficiency virus (HIV): This is a virus that can be passed through sexual contact with the vagina or anus, intravenous drug use, and blood transfusion. It can damage the immune system and raise the risk of contracting other viruses or bacteria and developing certain cancers. If left untreated, HIV can lead to acquired immunodeficiency syndrome (AIDS). But with pre-exposure prophylaxis (PrEP) as well as treatment after an HIV-positive diagnosis, many people living with HIV don't ever develop AIDS. In the early or acute stages, it's easy to mistake the symptoms of HIV for those of the flu.

Contraception

One of the biggest decisions your son can face is not whether to have sex, but when. Besides the emotional maturity required of intimacy, a big part of that decision also involves protection from infections or an unplanned pregnancy. Here is an overview of terms to help that conversation.

External condoms: Condoms are the only form of contraception that can reduce—but not completely eliminate—the risk of STIs and pregnancy during sex. If desired, you can make sure your son knows where to acquire/purchase condoms and how to put them on by visiting the FAQ and resources provided in the back of this book. There is no minimum age to buy condoms.

Internal condoms: The internal condom is inserted into the vagina or anus before sex to help prevent pregnancy and reduce the risk of STIs. An internal condom can be inserted up to two hours before penile-vaginal intercourse and is only good for one use. An internal condom and an external condom should never be used at the same time as they can easily break from the friction. Additionally, water-based lubricant is the only type of lube that should be used with condoms.

Short-term contraception: The pill, the patch, the ring, and the shot are all hormonal options that can reduce the risk of pregnancy. These allow an individual to have control over how often they get their period.

Long-term contraception: These methods include hormonal and nonhormonal options. An intrauterine device (IUD) must be inserted into the uterus by a qualified health-care provider, and can be taken out at any time. A nonhormonal IUD option called ParaGard is made of medical-grade copper and can prevent pregnancy for up to 12 years. An implant known as "the Rod" is inserted into your arm and can work for up to three years.

Emergency contraception: This is commonly known as the morning-after pill. This medication is taken by a uterus owner after penile-vaginal intercourse to reduce the risk of pregnancy if no protection was used or if other contraception failed. The brand Plan B can be purchased over the counter and must be taken within 72 hours of sex to be effective. Another brand known as Ella requires a prescription from a health-care provider and can be taken up to 120 hours after sex. Both should be taken as soon as possible after sex to be the most effective in blocking implantation of a fertilized egg in the uterus.

Abortion: Abortion is a legal method to end a pregnancy in the United States. You may have strong personal feelings for or against abortion, so be sure to talk to your son about your values and beliefs around this topic. Two types of abortion are available: a medication abortion and a surgical abortion. A medication abortion involves taking pills prescribed by a doctor that will terminate a pregnancy. A surgical abortion involves a procedure to remove the fetus from the uterus. Laws governing how old a person needs to be and whether they need a parent's permission to have an abortion vary from state to state.

STI Treatment and Prevention

There are a handful of effective medications that can treat and/or prevent certain STIs.

Pre-exposure prophylaxis, also known as PrEP, is a daily medication that reduces a person's risk of acquiring HIV before they are exposed to it. PrEP is for people who may have a higher risk of acquiring HIV. It requires a prescription from a health-care provider.

Post-exposure prophylaxis, also known as PEP, is a medication that can be taken up to 72 hours after sex to reduce the risk of acquiring HIV. The sooner PEP is taken after the sexual experience, the more effective it will be. PEP requires a prescription from a health-care provider.

Gardasil 9 helps protect individuals 9 to 45 years of age against the diseases caused by nine types of HPV. This includes cervical, vaginal, vulvar, and anal cancer; certain throat and back-of-mouth cancers; and genital warts.

Antibiotics treat and cure chlamydia, gonorrhea, and syphilis. They also require a prescription from a health-care provider.

Barrier protection is a general term that includes a number of different methods and practices. For example, dental dams prevent the mouth from coming into contact with the vagina, vulva, and anus. Barriers can help prevent the spread of herpes and chlamydia. Condoms cannot completely prevent the spread of these STIs.

KEEP IN MIND

- A strong sense of self enables your son to navigate the changes of adolescence and puberty.
- Gender identity is the way a person feels in regard to their own gender.
- Sexuality is the awareness, acceptance, and enjoyment of our own body and the bodies of others. Sexual orientation includes what causes us attraction and who/what we desire in relationships.
- Pronouns matter; gender and sexual identity/expression can vary.
- Decisions surrounding sexual wellness are all part of the human experience.

PART II

FOUNDATIONAL
PARENTING
STRATEGIES

Now that you have a solid grasp of the physical changes of puberty, as well as the social-emotional development during adolescence, let's move on to general approaches to connect with and care for your son. Topics will include encouraging conversation, trust, vulnerability, and emotional intimacy. This will be beneficial before we dive into specific parenting strategies related to sexual wellness in part III.

Each upcoming chapter will offer a real-world example from the life of an adolescent boy, case studies to encourage connections to your own parenting, or insight into scenarios your son may encounter. We will use them to illustrate practical guidelines and conversation starters for your personal use.

CHAPTER FOUR

Defining and Sharing Your Values

Before moving forward, it's important we focus on values and beliefs that guide and motivate our thoughts and actions. Part of developing through adolescence and into adulthood involves making decisions based on values rather than the reward/punishment motivations of childhood. Defining and sharing your values with your son will influence how he treats himself, how he interacts with others, and how he behaves in the world around him. In this chapter you'll find an expanded discussion on values, including an example to provide context, practical guidelines, and dialogue examples to help you facilitate your own discussions with your son.

Discover and Define

One of the most difficult things for a caregiver is to allow their child to live their own life. On paper, that sounds like a no-brainer—naturally we want our kids to grow up to create their own livelihood and be happy doing so. But we hold so much love for our young ones that in the moment we often just do things for them. It's a hard habit to break, given how much time we've spent providing food, clothes, shelter, and . . . well, everything.

Nevertheless, during adolescence we begin letting go of some of those duties. At the same time, we can prepare them for an independent life by teaching our children how to live according to household priorities and values. The delicate balance of parenthood includes instilling the morals that we believe in while allowing for our child's autonomous development. This means they will sometimes make decisions we don't value ourselves, whether it's a hobby or interest, or lifestyle choices such as careers and relationships.

Decisions aren't necessarily mistakes, however. You may disagree with something your child decides to pursue, but it still may be a valid choice for them. Certainly, if his values are illegal, harm himself, or harm others, that's another story. But if he's opting for another religion or declares he's vegan, and these are things that you don't value, you may need to engage in a healthy debate. Your positive influence matters, but in the end, it is his life. You might not make a certain life choice, but keep in mind your son is creating his own path.

So what are the values you want to pass on to your son? To help you articulate them, consider the categories below:

Character/Manners	Education	Work
Play	Family/Friends	Health
Finances	Spirituality/Mindfulness	Fun/Entertainment

For each of these, ask yourself:

"What's the main message I want to instill about this subject?" For example, relating to education, your message might be, "Finish schoolwork before recreational time."

"What do I hope my son comes to value in this area by adulthood?" For example, you might want your son to value creating stability and harmony with physical health, mental health, and social health.

"Are there specifics I can help with as he grows up?" On the topic of finances, you might teach your son how to manage a checking account. For good relationships with family and friends, you might teach him that communication takes active listening. Perhaps in establishing good manners, you'll explain that eye contact and a strong handshake are important when meeting someone.

Example

Eighth grader Jay (he/him) does well with his schoolwork, excels in track and field, and values time with friends. He does not agree with everything his parents value, however. Jay thinks his father is too controlling when it comes to religious service, and he thinks his mother is overly concerned with Jay's time spent playing video games. Jay believes he doesn't need such strict guidelines on weekends. Heading into high school, Jay begins complaining that he wants to stay out with his friends (mixed in gender) later on Saturday nights. He says his household has the earliest curfew time of his social group, and he's starting to feel isolated from them. Jay has said on more than one occasion that he wishes his parents were more like his friend Danny's (he/him)—they ask only that Danny text them so they won't wait up for him.

Practical Guidelines

Jay's story is an example of how considering a family's specific values can help create a path to resolution. If his mother has particular concerns about video games, it may help for her and Jay to discuss them and do some research to see how much caution is reasonable. On the other hand, the concern might be that video games are taking Jay's time away from other things, which is a whole different discussion. Some parents might be alarmed if, when pressed, Jay says that sometimes his friends do "hook up" with each other when they hang out after hours. Others might be relieved if Jay explains that he really doesn't care about that, and that for him it's just time to play games and goof around with his buddies. Getting at the values that are behind these kinds of conflicts can be more productive than arguing about curfews and permissions.

Here are a few considerations that can apply to sorting out differences in values:

Do no harm. Consider this major item to be the first and foremost priority in conflicts over values, beliefs, and traditions. In Jay's situation, is it possible for his parents to address their son's behavior without alienating him from his friends?

See the whole picture. Be an observer, willing to analyze events both worldwide and within the community through the lens of a parent. Jay's parents should take note if there are any events or activities in his social circle late at night that would put their son at risk. It would make sense for his caregiver to bring up religious history or current events that help connect to their belief system.

Start with why, then move to what. Teens and preteens appreciate knowing the reasoning behind things. This is certainly true with something as important as life values, and, in turn, customs and ethics. Why are sleep, safety, and screen time important values in Jay's family? Why do his parents want to keep tabs on him on weekends?

Keep things slow and steady. Small morsels of insight are plenty to help your son connect the dots himself. Jay's parents could prompt him to evaluate how keeping an early curfew helps him stay on top of his schoolwork and enables him to maintain consistent sleeping habits so he can get up early for track practice.

Your home, your call. Ultimately, as the parent, you have the final decision on household expectations set by your values. By all means, incorporate your son in the process and help him find his own values. But, frankly, he's not the parent. If you need to put your foot down and circle back to an argument days or even weeks down the line, so be it. However, make sure to follow up.

Open a Dialogue

As the caregiver, you may have your own values already established about certain aspects of puberty, relationships, and sexuality. Rest assured, there are ways to respect any boundaries you might have and still provide the best support for your son. Consistent conversations will help ease awkwardness, making future discussions that much easier. Here are some ways to communicate effectively about values.

> **Just start.** *Jump right into a conversation if you're not sure how to begin. "You know, I was thinking about life values a bit. Do you know some of the things we hold close to our heart as family priorities?"*
>
> **Use "I" statements.** *Avoid putting your son on the defensive. Instead of, "You drive me crazy when you're late like this!" try, "I'm frustrated right now because I thought we both valued being on time."*
>
> **Be straightforward.** *Hem and haw, and you may lose his attention before you make your point. "Hey, I wanted to follow*

up about Saturday night. What questions or complaints do you still have? I'm all ears."

Share an anecdote. *Draw attention to any appropriate personal examples. "I was struggling yesterday on where to spend my time, but I remembered I value ___ above ___."*

TAKEAWAYS

▸ Defining and sharing your values with your son will influence how he treats himself and interacts with the world.

▸ Values can include beliefs about things like education, work, play, manners, family/friends, health, and finances.

▸ Your son needs to become self-sufficient in carrying through with life values, making his own choices. You can plant the seed, provide warmth and water, but in the end you will need to step back and watch how things grow.

▸ To instill a sense of importance with values, be straightforward, keep things short, explain your reasoning, and use personal examples if they are appropriate.

CHAPTER FIVE

Establishing Mutual Trust and Respect

Chances are your son knows you as one of the first people in this world he *could* trust—in fact, he likely trusted you before he even knew what the word meant. But as with other matters, the turbulent changes of adolescence can put a new strain on that bond of trust, or at least make it feel less secure. In this chapter we'll explore how to establish, maintain, and deepen a connection of trust and respect with your son—one that will weather the storm as he transitions into maturity.

Discover and Define

The work you put in to maintain a level of understanding and reliability with your son will not only pay off in your bond with him, it will directly impact his ability and inclination to put trust in other people. The quality of his relationships with family, friends, and acquaintances will improve because of his experiences with you. And ultimately, his dating relationships will be more grounded in values and mutual trust.

You may not have given much thought to this, or maybe trust issues are a major concern at this point in your son's trajectory toward adulthood. Either way, it's helpful to evaluate the status quo by asking yourself: "In terms of trust, how do I want my relationship with my son to feel? What do respectful interactions with my son look and sound like, on both our parts?" Then consider how closely this matches what actually happens when the two of you communicate. Where do you see a need for a stronger bond? Are there specific situations in a typical week where you feel more trusting of him?

Next, look toward the future. Will your needs regarding trust change as your son ages? How? Is it time to start considering that next level of mutual trust? How will you know when the time comes?

Here are some specific aspects of trust to consider as you continue building respect with your son:

Responsibilities. Do you understand each other's weekly workload and duties?

Routines. Do you have the same default expectations for his whereabouts during a typical day or week?

Time frames. What do deadlines and leniency look like regarding schoolwork and chores?

Stressors. What tends to trigger disrespect or a break in trust? Are there ways to de-escalate those situations before damage is done?

Consequences. Is there consistency and fairness after misbehavior?

Expectations. When either of you has agreed to something, how often does the outcome match what is expected of you both?

Example

Amaan (he/him), a high school sophomore, has just learned to drive. His mother has only one car, and it's an older model that Amaan is a bit embarrassed about. Some of Amaan's friends have their own cars, but Amaan needs to work around his mom's job, as well as the activity schedule of his two younger siblings, to be able to drive. He's allowed access to the family car as long as he follows his mother's expectations: pay for his own gas (he earns money by working a summer job) and be home with the car before she needs to leave for work (she sometimes works evenings).

One Friday evening, Amaan stayed at a friend's house later than planned and brought the car home with an empty tank. Amaan's mother needed to stop for gas; she missed the beginning of her job shift and was reprimanded. When confronted about the incident, instead of apologizing Amaan blew up about how unfair it is that his friends all have their own cars and he has to beg for and borrow his mom's. Amaan stormed off to his room, screaming about never being able to ask anyone out on a date because he can never drive, and that he hates their ugly car anyway.

Practical Guidelines

As we noted in chapter two, adolescent boys are notorious for major mood swings. For the most part, they don't mean to hurt anyone. But their outbursts can strain the trust their caregivers put in them. It's common for a teen boy to lose an adult's trust with just one miscalculated decision that shatters the parent's image of their virtuous child. Take moments like these as reminders that your son isn't perfect, he's human. Try to see a lapse in respect for what it is: a misstep that calls for compassionate education. In Amaan's case, there's a lot going on that is deserving of a focused conversation—or, more likely, multiple conversations. Although it might be one stressor that triggers a teenage boy's rant, it's rarely just one thing in his world that causes such behavior.

From an outside perspective we might guess that Amaan's stress isn't just about the car. He may have other issues with his living conditions, or he may be feeling resentful of his more fortunate friends. That does not excuse his outburst, and it certainly does not allow him to break the agreement about the family car. But understanding this will help his mother address the larger issues.

Here are a few strategies that foster trust and respect between parent and child during adolescence:

Love unconditionally. Always remember to separate the behavior from the person. In Amaan's situation, his mother should address the timeliness issue first, and then examine ways to help his stress about the car, friends, and dating. She should not use the incident as a referendum on Amaan's character.

Give respect to earn respect. Maintaining a degree of respect even when your child has behaved badly or disappointed you doesn't make you foolish or permissive. It enables you to get to the root of the matter. Amaan's mother must temporarily look past her son's outburst and address where his hurt is coming from.

Once she sorts through that, it's time to explain the harm of his actions from her perspective.

Show that lost trust can be regained. Allow your son a second chance; you know that real life is full of them. But do be clear that it's increasingly more difficult to trust someone after a bond has been broken. In Amaan's case, his mother can decide to ground him and revoke his car privileges for a while until he builds up her trust again over the next few weeks by sticking to his chores, schoolwork, and other responsibilities.

Debate without blame. Hear your son's side of the story with an eye toward finding solutions rather than finding fault. Amaan's mother should ask her son if he has any ideas of how to help their collective cause. What if he drove her to work some nights and reimbursed her for a rideshare to bring her home?

Open a Dialogue

In order to talk about trust issues with your adolescent, you may be able to simply dive in to discuss what's happening while it's actually happening. However, more than likely it will take a little bit of cunning, and possibly extra time, to crack open a solid conversation. This is especially true if your son tends to be quiet and reserved, or if he treats your discussions like lectures.

Try these opening gambits:

> **Give fair warning.** *"Hey bud, you and I need to have a quick chat about the other night. I'll be around at lunchtime today. Let's clear some things up then, okay?"*

> **Provide movement.** *"Hey, let's talk while you help me drag those boxes from the garage to the curb."*

Hold your end of the deal. *"I know I said you would be able to use the car tonight, and you can. But you didn't tell me you were driving out of town, so here's how it's going to work."*

When in doubt, try food. *"I'm hungry. You? Let's go grab some food, just the two of us, and figure out how you can earn the money you owe your mother."*

Begin—and end—on a high note. *"I love you, you know. That will never, ever change."*

TAKEAWAYS

- The work you put in to maintain a level of understanding and reliability with your son will directly impact his trust in others.
- Considerations for building respect and mutual trust include responsibilities, routines, time frames, stressors, consequences, and expectations.
- Adolescents often test parental trust, but try to see disrespect as a misstep in need of compassionate education. Separate the behavior from the person, and love unconditionally.
- For big talks, a heads-up is nice so your son doesn't feel defensive. Make it the same day to avoid dread. For short chats, walks-and-talks might work well, or, as clichéd as it sounds, try a game of catch or something similar.

CHAPTER SIX

Facilitating Openness

Openness refers to the willingness to experience new things and to share in the varying experiences of others. It's a key attribute for adolescent boys who are beginning to pursue independent experiences. Openness affects how they encounter and understand differing cultures, customs, and traditions, as well as how they act and react in social settings. To be open is not to automatically accept everyone's opinion, but rather to avoid knee-jerk judgment and to consider different points of view. It's a posture that facilitates lifelong learning, kindness, and empathy. As a caregiver, you will want to model a positive outlook on the diversity of ideas and lifestyles that your son will come across not just in his youth, but throughout his life. In the following pages we'll highlight how you can cultivate this kind of outlook as your maturing son turns his attention to a wider world.

Discover and Define

As an adult, you might find openness a simple concept to understand. But do all adults put it into practice? We all fall into the trap of being calcified in our opinions and automatically rejecting whatever makes us uncomfortable. Merely stating the importance of openness won't have as much impact on your son as demonstrating the merit of exploring diverse viewpoints. Here are some subjects that can spark those kinds of discussions:

Family heritage and traditions. If you know your lineage, what kinds of things were previous generations of your family doing when they were your son's age?

Cultural traditions. What kinds of rituals or traditions does your culture have for adolescents? What's the meaning behind them? Do they feel relevant? What traditions feel uncomfortable to you that you could share with your son?

National and world history. Either in person or through the power of websites, you can explore landmarks, monuments, museums, plays, and concerts that hold different meanings for different groups.

Politics and political parties. Parents can share nonpartisan global issues that help expand their son's worldview and, in turn, his openness to varied personal relationships, like friendships and dating interests.

Food, art, sports, and entertainment. Build a habit of trying new experiences with your son—a different cuisine when dining out, a trip to an offbeat museum, a webcast of sports competitions from other countries. Even if some of these turn out to be duds, being open to new experiences is a prelude to healthy vulnerability and emotional intimacy in romantic relationships.

In addition, encourage your son to open up about the following personal topics:

School routines. With a preteen, ask about locker issues, traveling to class, or note-taking; for an older teen, ask about workload balance or project completion. At any age, help your son examine his study time and techniques. Ask him directly, "How do you plan on studying for that big test this week?" Open communication about something as benign as school helps in the trickier communication about dating relationships and intimacy.

Physical boundaries or injuries. Help your son get comfortable asking for personal space by being forthright: "Hey, can you back up a little? I'm feeling crowded here." Reinforce how healthy it is to reach out for help if injured in a game or during play. This is practice for moving through embarrassment while being direct with other private issues of puberty like hygiene, shaving, or underwear needs.

Social discomfort and peer pressure. Commend basic openness about uncomfortable social scenarios, like being expected to share homework or feeling pressured to exclude someone from a group night out. Assist your son in these situations by applauding his assessment of that "off" feeling he has when something is not right. This social recognition connects to consent—an essential for any safe and pleasurable intimate relationship.

Example

High schooler Ry (they/them) is an intelligent and conscientious, albeit shy, teenager. They tell their parents that some friends are involved in social justice causes, using media platforms to promote awareness and education on important issues. Ry feels a strong desire to participate, but just doesn't get how their friends can put themselves out there. Ry feels embarrassed to do so without having all the facts on a subject. Ry has been to rallies and marches endorsing human equality and equity but is cautious about seeming more committed to the ideas than they actually are. It's also true that Ry's afraid of criticism. Ry is so sensitive about being wrong that they often don't act at all.

Practical Guidelines

Ry's parents can point out that openness to new experiences includes comfort with the possibility of things not going the way you want them to and the prospect of making mistakes. There's no mandate for Ry to step outside their comfort zone, but if Ry really wants the experience of being more socially involved, they'll have to risk failing. If things don't go well, they can analyze what happened and learn from it—that, too, is a reward of openness. Some adolescents need to be cautioned about jumping heedlessly into the fray. But others may need to be reminded that too much fear of doing the wrong thing can be stultifying and rob them of valuable life experience.

Here are a few considerations for nurturing an open mindset in an earnest adolescent:

Explain the benefits. Ry might find that risking new experiences is beneficial in unexpected ways. There's a strong correlation between having an accepting worldview and having a healthy social life. When you reject all unfamiliar concepts, your pool of potential friends shrinks considerably. An attitude of openness also has a positive effect on mental and emotional well-being.

Relate examples. Share tales from your family heritage about risks taken, new ideas embraced, and relationships forged with unlikely compatriots. Perhaps Ry's parents were activists themselves in their younger days. If your ancestry is unknown, research stories from history, especially involving times and places your son is interested in.

Explore multiple points of view. Don't shy away from the dark times of human existence. Use age-appropriate renditions of historical events to help your son understand that there are diverse stories to be told, and that not all of them get the attention they deserve. Or follow up on news reports to explore how marginalized and underrepresented groups are affected.

Open a Dialogue

Start conversations and discussions with these strategic moves:

Tell a story. *Share your own direct accounts of witnessing empathy and openness within the family. "Did you ever hear about the time your grandmother joined a civil rights march and got arrested?"*

Compliment empathy. *"I noticed you shoveled the neighbor's sidewalk this morning. I'm so proud that you'd help a senior without being asked. You care deeply about your community, and it shows."*

Label advocacy. *Point out advocacy, and self-advocacy, by using these terms when your son gets involved. "I heard you on the phone with your friend, advocating for the homeless who are being harassed by the police. Impressive! Can you tell me more about that cause?"*

TAKEAWAYS

- Openness can be inspired and encouraged through stories—both those that are relatable and those that introduce new cultures and concepts. Adolescents benefit from both.
- Parents can prompt growth in their son's self-awareness and social appreciation through conversations that draw attention to acceptance.
- Encourage openness by helping your son advocate and self-advocate. Identifying, representing, and communicating one's own needs—as well as those of others—are skills that will be used in closer intimate relationships later in life.

CHAPTER SEVEN

Embracing Vulnerability

We often associate vulnerability with weakness, and nobody likes to admit to being weak—especially adolescent boys. But vulnerability has a positive context: acknowledging difficult emotions instead of avoiding or repressing them. We can think of vulnerability as the next step progressing from openness. Where openness is a willingness to experience new things and celebrate diversity in others, vulnerability turns that attitude inward, acknowledging our full self and admitting to our faults, fears, and limitations.

Vulnerability is authenticity, particularly when circumstances call for real, emotional responses. In this sense, vulnerability is not weakness, but rather the contrary; vulnerability takes strength and confidence. Becoming comfortable with discomfort, both on your part and the part of your son, will help with conversations about relationships and sexual wellness. In this chapter we'll discuss the value of vulnerability and see how you can support it in your son and in yourself.

Discover and Define

Vulnerability is useful. Yet it needs to be harnessed correctly. As a caregiver, your own maturity is an important asset for helping your adolescent son acknowledge and develop vulnerability.

That's because in order to help your son with the courage to be vulnerable to himself and to others in his life, you'll also need to embrace vulnerability yourself. Being vulnerable involves uncertainty and perhaps a risk that feels uncomfortable. Fortunately, as an adult, you've done this often, because every parent needs to admit their limits and ask for help at some point. Just by picking up this book, you're doing it once again.

To assist your son's journey into a healthy, rewarding relationship with himself, leading to fulfilling, pleasurable relationships with others, you will need to admit a few things—first to yourself, and then potentially to him. Below are some difficult questions for you to reflect on. Attempt some initial responses without overthinking, then mull things over a bit during the course of a day or week. Revisit as often as needed.

What do you fear about parenting an adolescent?

How does your upbringing impact your parenting style?

What conversation topics bring you the most discomfort?

What life changes did you dread? What life changes weren't as bad as you thought? Were any of them worse?

Do you have any guilty pleasures? Why are you guilty about them?

What emotion(s) do you tend to cover up?

What weakness(es) (personality, skill, or otherwise) do you consider embarrassing?

Who has had an overwhelmingly positive impact on your life? Is there anyone you would qualify as having the opposite effect?

What comment(s), either positive or negative, do you hold on to from years past?

When have you disappointed someone? When have you disappointed yourself?

Do you hide any behavior(s), even minor habits, from people?

When, where, and what have you given up on? Did it bother you? Does it now?

What seems easy for everybody but you?

In what situation(s) did you exhibit courage in life?

Example

Isaac (he/him) is 12 years old and lives with his parents and grand-mother. He has always been close to his friends growing up, some of whom have been into sports, some into gaming, and others into art and music. Isaac likes the variety, but he only recently shared his interest in photography with his good friend Leena (she/her). She doesn't know much about photography, but she likes drawing and animation. They both enjoy the time with each other and discussing new projects. Isaac wishes he could share this creative side of himself with some of his other friends, but he thinks they won't care, or worse—that they might make fun of him. Leena has repeatedly offered that she can be right next to him if/when he wants to open up.

Practical Guidelines

Here are some principles to follow when discussing and supporting vulnerability in your child:

Listen first. As the parent, refrain from interjecting too early, or too often, when your son shares information about what's going on in his life. Allow your teenage boy to work out when, and what, to share with you. Remember that deep conversations require more than one side; cultivate your own awareness and compassion, and save your input for the right time so you don't unwittingly dominate a conversation. Hear your son out—which is sometimes all that is needed—and then assist where possible.

Reserve judgment. Don't rush to fight his battles. The important thing is that he's comfortable enough in your relationship to be vulnerable with you. Isaac's caregivers might not believe exposing his interest in photography is that big a deal, but telling him that won't be helpful. Instead, they can be mindful of helping him be his authentic self—without doing the work for him.

Caution him against oversharing. Vulnerability is not just letting the dam break on any and all personal information. The flow of vulnerability can be tough to get going, but once started, it can be even more difficult to stop. Although respecting Isaac's privacy, his caregivers can try to witness how he eventually communicates his interests with friends, over the phone perhaps, or on social media. They can offer gentle suggestions if he seems to be overdoing it. The same applies to your son. Reel him in as needed.

Honor his boundaries. Although oversharing is a concern, it's also true that being vulnerable can establish further boundaries. Vulnerability involves speaking our truth—what we want, need, and deserve. It's not an obligation to share everything. Respect how far your son is willing to go when opening up to you and be wary of pushing this comfort level too far. Let him know that others should show him the same respect.

Let down your defenses. When vulnerable, we are open to hurt. When hurt, we retaliate or shut down. Model healthy vulnerability to your son by staying open to his constructive criticism, even if it's hard to hear. Isaac's caregivers can help him see that letting down his defenses is potentially the most difficult yet most mature step in using vulnerability to his advantage for an authentic life.

Open a Dialogue

An important principle regarding vulnerability: Above all else, aim for authenticity. Your goal isn't a simulation or forced vulnerability that will probably omit self-reference. Rather than pushing vulnerability on your son to get something, allow it to naturally occur in order to help something. For example:

Help your son see through the social "masks" that others wear. *"Looking back to when I was in school, I now realize people covered up their true selves. Do you see any of that? When? Why?"*

Come right out with a question, if the mood fits. *"I know you're having trouble with your geometry class. How does it feel when you get a low score on a test?"*

Praise his courage. *Positive praise can bring more appropriate vulnerability in the future. "I noticed you were your true self when you admitted to your friend you're too scared of heights to try rock climbing. I'd be proud of admitting that . . . were you? Did it feel scary to say so?"*

TAKEAWAYS

▶ Vulnerability means acknowledging difficult emotions instead of avoiding or repressing them.

▶ Vulnerability is useful, if harnessed correctly. As a parent, being vulnerable with yourself can help you understand how to help your son do the same.

▶ Listen, reserve judgment, set boundaries, and, above all else, aim for authenticity. Vulnerability builds on openness to lead to peace, happiness, belonging, and emotional/sexual intimacy.

CHAPTER EIGHT

Encouraging Emotional Intimacy

Intimacy, in basic terms, refers to the closeness between people who feel safe and secure with one other. But intimacy is much more than that, of course. Every relationship is surrounded by a unique set of circumstances, so in the end every intimate interaction is one of a kind. For adolescent boys, it can be challenging to figure out how intimacy fits with ideas of maleness, especially because intimacy is so derided by messages of toxic masculinity in the wider culture. You can help your son navigate these waters by understanding where he's at in his social relationships, modeling the value of intimacy yourself, and being available to offer counsel or just hear his concerns. Let's take a look at how that works.

Discover and Define

We want adolescent boys to know that whatever level of connection they experience with someone can be normal. Their ability to connect will change and deepen as they develop more capacity for care, communication, and commitment. Timelines are always tricky, but here's a typical progression:

Around ages 9 to 11, boys might start to show independence from family and increased interest in friends.

Around ages 10 to 14, boys tend to begin spending more time in mixed gender groups, which could lead to crushes or dating relationships.

Around ages 15 to 19, friendships tend to become deeper and more stable, whereas romantic relationships can become central to a boy's social life.

Below is a list of a few common qualities that denote intimacy in a relationship, though not all need to be present since each relationship is unique. This list is not exhaustive; consider including what you as the parent would deem important qualities to add.

Care	Communication	Commitment	Collaboration	Time Together
Similar Values	Mutual Trust	Openness	Vulnerability	Humor
Shared Interests	Knowledge of Home Life	Reliability	Routines/ New Experiences	Empathy

It's also important to know the signs that intimacy is lacking. Without emotional intimacy in a relationship, your son might feel:

embarrassed	insulted
frustrated	betrayed
defensive	unheard or unacknowledged
misunderstood	
overly competitive	unwanted or unfulfilled
left alone	uneasy or unsafe
picked on	

To help your son—and you—assess the intimacy in any given relationship, ask about a few of these concepts during a conversation about a friend or partner. (The lists work for both friendships and dating.) Absence of positive qualities and overabundance of negative ones could be a sign that the relationship isn't healthy and needs to be repaired or brought to an end. If the converse is true, that may help your son appreciate the value of the friendship or connection.

Example

Felipe (he/him) and Ace (they/them) are both 17 years old and in a dating relationship. They've had deep conversations over where their relationship is headed once high school is over and they're each attending college in other states. After questioning what the future brings, they mutually decide they'll make their relationship open and agree to see other people. Felipe is working through the difficulties of this, however, because he would like to see the two of them try to stay exclusively committed and make the distance work. Felipe has not expressed this to Ace, worrying it will push Ace further away.

Practical Guidelines

What should parents do to encourage emotional intimacy and support their adolescent through life's peaks and valleys? Here are some options.

Encourage openness, vulnerability, and collaboration. Intimacy involves an invitation through words and actions. Essentials to intimacy include care, communication, and commitment, all of which take collaboration. Felipe and his caregivers can collectively brainstorm ways for him to express his connection to Ace by sharing academic and extracurricular activities with them.

Urge a balance in communication styles. Some texting and social media communication can benefit intimate relationships. Key word: some. Although apart, adolescents still want to feel connected to friends, particularly with crushes or while dating. But too much of either online or in-person interaction, depending on the relationship, can have the opposite effect on emotional intimacy. In Felipe's case, shifting the balance more toward texting and online video may help him feel better about the upcoming distanced communication with Ace.

Affirm feelings and experiences. Instead of attempting to solve your son's problems, or him trying to solve the problems of others, you both should remember that simply being present and listening is considerate and affirming. Such empathy benefits the listener's mental health, too.

Stay in their corner. Intimacy involves being a reliable ally. Even through disagreement, you are always rooting for your son. Felipe's caregivers might prefer he date other people rather than have an exclusive partner at his age. But understanding his pain, they can simply state, and restate, their unconditional love for him.

Embrace closeness and accept loss. Emotional intimacy can come and go along with the relationships themselves. Remind your son that we should be mindful of how fortunate we are to share closeness when a relationship is at its height, but that we must also stay grounded if it crashes.

Open a Dialogue

Intimacy can occur in any relationship with communication and closeness. It does not need to be romantic or sexual in nature. Intimacy can occur with platonic friends just as it can with love interests. At the onset of dating, intimacy may only be in its infancy, at least for those who have just met. In the case of friends turned more-than-friends, a high level of emotional intimacy may already be present. Both ways, and everything in between, can create fulfillment. Help your son comprehend all this in your discussions.

> **Begin with care.** *Vulnerability leads to relinquishing control or total knowledge of a situation. Start by simply showing care about the relationship your son is focusing on and not presuming anything. "So what's up with you? Are you seeing anyone?"*

> **Encourage openness.** *Think about the ways you can pose a question that will allow your son to open up a bit. "If you're looking for closeness, have you tried more time together? What things are you doing to stay in daily communication with them while they're away during the break?"*

> **Discuss details.** *Increased time together and practice with communication synthesize for a deeper connection in a relationship. But your son may need help finding ways to make that happen. "Relationships are certainly not jobs, but they do involve some work to maintain them. What routines do you two have? What new things do you try together?"*

TAKEAWAYS

- Intimacy is a safe closeness. It can occur in any relationship that features care, communication, and commitment.
- Each relationship is unique. Help your son know that whatever level of connection he experiences can be normal.
- Positive intimacy traits include similar values, trust, openness, and appropriate vulnerability.
- Affirm your son's feelings and experiences with intimacy. Instead of solving any problems that come up, simply remain present and in his corner.
- Intimacy takes time. Just like your connection with your son, the comfort he has with others requires a bit of work to both begin and maintain.

PART III

SPECIFIC SEXUAL HEALTH STRATEGIES FOR BOYS

In the previous chapters of this book, we've reviewed puberty changes, addressed masculinity, examined social and emotional issues, explored values and trust, and wrestled with vulnerability and intimacy. In the chapters ahead, you'll see how that established knowledge base will enable you to call upon specific scenarios and strategies regarding sexual health. Statistics, case studies, and sample dialogues will empower you as a caregiver to guide your child through delicate but necessary topics such as dating, consent, safe sex, pornography, and being a considerate ally to others.

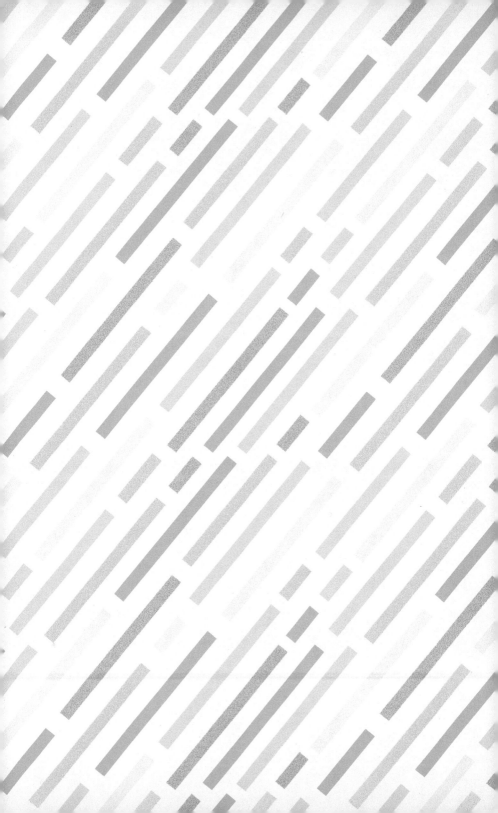

CHAPTER NINE

Nurturing Healthy Dating Relationships

Dating relationships in adolescence are about figuring out romantic intimacy. Teens are working through how to get from initial attraction to eventual love, which won't necessarily happen with the same person. Growing up, our sons practice sports skills, musical scales, and foreign language vocabulary. And in dating, they practice romantic love. Contrary to the well-worn aphorism, practice does not make perfect. But practice matters.

In the following pages, we'll look at some realities of teen romance and review some key considerations that impact your son's dating life.

Background and Considerations

Teen relationships can originate from a few types of attraction. Before your son has any desire to date, crushes tend to turn up on his radar. These can come in the form of an identity crush—that is, becoming fascinated by someone he admires and wants to follow or imitate. More familiarly, he might develop a romantic crush, finding someone attractive enough to want more than a friendship.

You can nurture your son's maturation process by asking what he finds attractive in his crush, even if it's an infatuation with a celebrity or someone he's unlikely to meet in real life. Help your son see what characteristics he might potentially look for in a future partner, focusing on attributes that are deeper than surface-level attractions. As he ages into his upper teen years, make this emphasis increasingly obvious, so he learns to appreciate people for more than physical looks.

Crushes and attractions generally show up by the middle school/junior high school years. Parents can plan on hearing about dating relationships by ages 13 to 14. Sometimes younger teens will "see" or "go out" with someone for just a few days. This is typical. Avoid being too nosy or too judgmental about the brevity of dating relationships. Remember, adolescents are practicing intimacy here. Disparaging comments and terms like "puppy love" can downplay the importance of learning how to date.

Teenagers will vary in how much intimacy they desire and how many relationships they pursue. Dating can help teens find out what they require to avoid loneliness, as well as how much closeness they can tolerate before feeling saturated.

It is helpful to know a few facts about teen romance:

Around 66 percent of teenagers have been in at least one dating relationship in the last 12 months.

Teens ages 15 to 17 are around twice as likely as those ages 13 to 14 to have had a romantic relationship in the last year (44 percent vs. 20 percent).

Older teens are more likely to say they are currently in an active relationship, serious or otherwise (18 percent vs. 6 percent of younger teens).

The average dating relationship at ages 12 to 14 lasts less than five months. For ages 15 to 18, the average is less than two years.

Estimates are that fewer than 5 percent of teen relationships become a committed adult romance.

Example

Evan (he/him) is 16 years old and finally dating a classmate whom he's had a crush on for almost two years. They've only been dating for about a month, but the two of them have been close friends for a while, and Evan is excited to see where things go. He really likes his partner's sense of humor and shared interests, in addition to their physical looks. The pair holds hands, cuddles during movies, and have kissed during a few make out sessions. Evan makes nightly phone calls to talk. For Valentine's Day, Evan picked up some flowers and treats, proud to bring them to school with a thoughtfully written card. The gifts were met with a curt, almost embarrassed response; Evan's significant other did not get him anything in return. In fact, Evan felt avoided all day. When he brought it up after school, emotionally hurt and worried, Evan's partner did exactly what he dreaded: They broke up with him. It was abrupt and without argument. Evan's ex explained that they tried the relationship because of their great connection—plus, friends nudged it to become official—but they eventually felt a bit suffocated and didn't see them working out as more than friends.

Practical Guidelines

In Evan's scenario, we might see that neither teen was in the wrong. The two of them had different expectations, which perhaps could have been communicated, but the relationship was pursued for what seems like the right reasons.

Adolescents may seek a dating relationship with a person who we, as the parent, can tell might not be that interested in our son. But that kind of mismatch is part of the learning process, a chance for adolescents to find out who to pursue for a relationship and how to form an intimate connection together. This isn't to say parents shouldn't intervene if things seem unsafe or blatantly unhealthy, but making mistakes is how young people learn, even with intimacy. Disappointment and heartbreak, although unfortunate, can build resilience and create clarity for closer connections in the future.

Here are a few specific considerations for nurturing adolescent dating relationships:

Don't put pressure in either direction. To date or not to date? Let your son decide when he's ready. Dating relationships offer the potential for personal growth, such as Evan learning about his own needs and desires and gaining experience with complex emotions. On the other hand, some teens who don't date report less stress, anxiety, or depression, and they sometimes exhibit better social skills compared to their dating peers.

Be cautious with labels. If your son is dating someone, he will most likely stay away from applying the word "love" to the situation, at least for a while. The term can be scary for anyone, most particularly the typical teenager. Expect to hear boyfriend, girlfriend, or a nonbinary endearment like "the person I'm seeing/dating" or "my partner." When in doubt, just call them friends.

Brace for breakups. They happen. Breakups are a major reality of teen dating. In adulthood, once a dating relationship passes the one-year mark, statistics for breakups decrease. This isn't true for teenagers; up to 95 percent of teen relationships will end. Remind your son that a breakup doesn't mean the relationship was a waste of time.

Give him points for being vulnerable. Getting your heart broken takes vulnerability. Even being the one to end things can be revelatory. It's important to respect whatever emotional journey occurs through your son's sadness and anger into acceptance and hope. Evan's caregivers supported their son before and during the dating process, but their greatest effort might come in helping him after the breakup. They can lead by commending him on being vulnerable enough to put himself out there in the first place.

Open a Dialogue

Here are some potential questions that can help your son make decisions about whether or not to date:

Does he have a sense of self before or outside of a dating relationship? *Ask, "What habits or characteristics do you want to maintain, regardless of relationship status?"*

Where does dating fit into current priorities? *Ask, "Will you be able to keep up with school/sports/music/art, etc.?"*

What rationale is there to date or stay single? *Ask, "Would you date because you genuinely like the person, or just for social appearances? What are you worried about, if anything, about being in a relationship?"*

Communicate relationship expectations. *Ask, "Are you satisfied with the level of intimacy in the relationship? Do you see a near future with this significant other?"*

Explain that breakups can also occur when teens spend too much time together. *Ask, "Do you feel like you have personal time and space? Can you effectively manage time apart, if it comes to that?"*

Upon a breakup, encourage your son to focus on sleep, exercise, meditation—whatever healthy practices seem to work for him. *Say, "Hey bud, I'm thinking of you. Take some time alone for a while. I'll check back on you in two hours and we'll all go to dinner."*

TAKEAWAYS

- Dating relationships in adolescence are about figuring out romantic intimacy. Practice with dating is practice with romantic love.
- Around 66 percent of teenagers have been in at least one dating relationship in the last 12 months.
- Like adults, teenagers will vary in how much intimacy they desire and how many relationships they pursue.
- Both dating and not dating can have benefits for teens.
- Breakups happen. Getting your heart broken takes vulnerability.

CHAPTER TEN

Instilling a Comprehensive Understanding of Consent

Consent is the permission for something to happen; it is actively agreeing to an activity. In a relationship, consent involves both individuals agreeing upon the same thing. Specifically, sexual consent is an agreement between participants to engage in sexual contact.

As we continue to build specific sexual health strategies for parents, consent will be one of our top criteria for teens to have safe and pleasurable relationships. We want adolescent boys to fully comprehend consent, beginning with emotional connections and continuing through any sexual activity. Consent communicates values and facilitates intimacy. It is respect, openness, and vulnerability in action. Consent shows love.

With this chapter, we'll share some important facts, concepts, and considerations related to consent and how to pass these messages to your son.

Background and Considerations

Consent is necessary because a person's body is their property. Whether dating or not, giving and getting permission to have physical contact is always needed. Your son's safety and satisfaction depend on knowing that consent means he's not being pressured to do something, especially an activity he doesn't want to do. Equally important, it means he must not pressure anyone, romantic and sexual partners included, into doing anything, either. Consent feels right because it creates comfort and respect for everyone. And that's just what a developing gentleman should aim for.

Consent also equates to self-respect. Your son is in charge of deciding if and when anyone gets to touch him, and that is empowering when entering the dating world. He can agree, or disagree, to something as simple as holding hands to something more intimate like kissing or sexual touch. Likewise, the person he's with has the same entitlement.

The principle of consent includes significant legal consequences when it comes to sexual matters. Sexual consent laws vary by nation, state, and sometimes community. In some cases, even consensual sexual activity in which one or both individuals are below a certain age—the legal "age of consent"—is considered a criminal act. Be sure to have a frank discussion with your son about the applicable laws in your area.

One way to impart the meaning of consent is to use the acronym **FRIES**. Consent is always:

Freely given: Each choice should be made without pressure, manipulation, or the influence of drugs or alcohol.

Reversible: Anyone can change their mind at any time about what they feel like doing, even in the middle of an activity.

Informed: Someone can only consent to something if they have the full story. Lies and deceit cannot lead to consent.

Enthusiastic: In a relationship, consent is doing things as desired. Activities should not be done because they're expected; they should be welcome and fun.

Specific: Saying yes to one thing in a relationship does not mean someone is saying yes to other actions, even if they've done them before.

In our discussion about masculinity in chapter two, we noted the societal messages about manhood can conflict with the idea of respectful, consensual interaction. Your son may wonder why you feel the need to ensure that he understands consent. Here are some numbers that illustrate that respect for consent is not a universal virtue and should be actively championed. (Warning: Included are triggering descriptions and statistics about sexual violence.)

- About 16 percent of adult women and 3 percent of adult men have reported being the victim of an attempted or completed rape in their lifetime.
- An estimated 15 percent of sexual assault victims are ages 12 to 17. About 82 percent of all juvenile victims are female.
- Among the teenagers who reported dating during the previous 12 months, 8 percent experienced dating and/or sexual violence.
- Around 21 percent of transgender, genderqueer, or gender-nonconforming college students have reported being sexually assaulted.

(Note: See the Resources section in the back of this book if you need support or more information regarding sexual assault or violence.)

Example

Matt (he/him) and Kayla (she/her) have been dating for exactly one year. They have participated in some sexual touching but have never had sexual intercourse. After a nice dinner and a movie, they start to make out. Matt tells Kayla that since it's their one-year anniversary, if she really loves him, she would have sex with him. Kayla verbally expresses her hesitance but does enjoy kissing and touching. She also loves Matt and doesn't want to lose him. While the make out session continues, Matt initiates oral sex on Kayla, who goes silent. Matt interprets Kayla's silence as a sign that she's into it. They proceed to have oral sex, which leads to intercourse. Throughout, Kayla doesn't say no to anything, but she doesn't say yes, either.

Practical Guidelines

In Matt and Kayla's case, the sexual behavior was nonconsensual. Applying the FRIES criteria, we see that those elements were almost completely missing. Kayla could and should report the incident to authorities as sexual assault, even if she does have a romantic relationship with Matt. In the aftermath, counseling will be necessary for both individuals, particularly for Kayla to realize she was not in the wrong and should never blame herself in any way.

It is critical to pass the messages of consent on to your son during discussions of intimacy. To combat the perpetuation of rape culture, combine consent talks with an examination and critique of toxic masculinity, media messages, and pornography. Sexual assault is never the victim's fault, no matter the situation, reputation, clothing, substance use, flirting, or foreplay involved. Be relentless in calling out victim-blaming in media or real-life scenarios, pointing out to your son the harm that apologist behavior causes.

Here are a few specific considerations for helping your son incorporate consent into every relationship.

Start early. Opportunities for teaching your son about consent are available well before he enters adolescence, let alone dating or sexual relationships. For very young kids, adults can instill a sense of consent without even mentioning the term. While tickling them, for example, draw attention to words like "stop," "don't," or "no more" that bring the behavior to an end. This demonstrates respect for one's body. With young teens and preteens, moments like wrestling, roughhousing, or affectionate verbal teasing can also serve this purpose. Cease the teasing with a mention like, "Notice I stopped when you said 'Stop!' That's kind, right?" When roles are reversed, highlight consent once again: "I'm proud of how you listened and reacted to the word 'no.' That's known as consent." Quick, simple, and effective moments like this will weave the concept into their way of thinking.

Emphasize the finality of no. "No" doesn't mean "convince me." Communication during sexual contact might include negotiation, but not in the sense of pleading or making deals. Negotiation in intimacy means finding a common ground, not convincing the other to accept your terms. Your son should know he might hear "no" more than "yes," and that's perfectly acceptable. It's also worth explaining that affirmative consent may never happen with a specific someone or with regard to a particular activity. This also demands respect and compliance on the other partner's part. Consent is a never-ending consideration for intimate relationships.

Establish a precedent. Hugs and kisses from relatives are often expected. But physical touch in any relationship is always an individual's decision. Pushing a child into an embrace, even with a loved one, can send conflicting messages about their body. As soon as your child is able to voice an opinion, offer them other options, like a high-five or a wave. Children may eventually choose affection on their own, and by the teen years parents can then underline the power of "no" and the power of "yes."

Explain that no answer is not an answer. Matt should have immediately noticed that Kayla's behavior was not enthusiastic. His purported needs were put ahead of Kayla's, and there was never clear, enthusiastic consent involved. The absence of no does not imply yes.

Open a Dialogue

Accepting no for an answer during a date does not put a halt on intimacy or wreck the relationship. Here's some language your son can use for discussing consent while maintaining affection.

"Do you want to get closer?"

"Not now. I'm just gonna lean my head on you like this."

"Yeah, sounds good. I'm also up for more if you change your mind."

"We can make out later tonight, maybe. We'll see."

"Cool. No rush. If it doesn't happen that's okay, too."

"Thanks. Past kissing, I'm not comfortable yet, though. You?"

"Agreed. Just being with you is nice."

It bears repeating that the absence of "no" does not imply "yes." Even in the heat of the moment, working toward enthusiastic sexual consent won't ruin things. Some easy ways to assess consent include:

"Are you comfortable?"

"What do you like?"

"Is this okay?"

"Do you want to slow down?"

"Do you want to go any further?"

"Are you still okay with this?"

"Are you sure?"

TAKEAWAYS

- Consent is the permission for something to happen. It is actively agreeing to an activity and must be freely given, reversible, informed, enthusiastic, and specific.
- Consent cannot be implied by silence or obtained by force or pressure. Saying nothing, or saying yes while under the influence of drugs or alcohol, is not consent.
- Your son is in charge of deciding if and when anyone gets to touch him, and whoever he's with has the same privilege.

CHAPTER ELEVEN

Exploring Safer Sex

As we described in the very beginning of this book, imparting sex positivity—the mindset that sexuality is a natural, healthy, pleasurable part of the human experience—is critical for your son's sex education. But that doesn't mean that sexuality never includes making carefully considered choices or acting responsibly. The term "safe sex" may seem to imply danger or risk. But what it really refers to is making informed, personal decisions that match one's desires for emotional and physical intimacy while safeguarding the well-being of everyone involved. This can include using protective methods to lower the risk of sexually transmitted infections and having knowledge about and access to contraception to prevent unwanted pregnancy. In this chapter, we'll equip you to help your son make the choices that will keep him safe while maintaining a sex-positive message that he can connect with.

Background and Considerations

Whatever your own beliefs about sex and virginity, if you're like many parents, you'd likely breathe a sigh of relief if your son opted for abstinence as the safest sexual choice during adolescence. But what happens if that isn't the case? Do you have a plan? Not everyone in their teenage years wants to sexually abstain, particularly since sex is a healthy part of an intimate relationship. This is particularly pertinent for parents of older teens, but every caregiver needs to plant the seed ahead of time that sex should be enjoyable but *safe*.

Along with that recommendation, be certain to focus your values on consent and pleasure instead of fear and shame. Safe sex is pleasurable sex, after all. And putting a positive angle on teen behavior receives more consideration than berating them with what not to do. Imagine the constant message of doom your son receives from all directions: "Don't eat junk food. Don't stay up too late. Don't drive too fast. Don't drink. Don't do drugs. Don't have sex." Teens might think, "Well, I've had my share of soda and candy, and I'm okay. Same when I stay up late. Plus, Dad speeds all the time. And Mom drinks wine at dinner." Adding sex to the long list of things not to do makes it an easy message to ignore.

Let's look at some numbers to help understand trends with adolescent sexual contact, as background for discussions with your son. At the time of publication:

- Around 38 percent of teenagers have had sexual contact.
- Older teens are more likely to be sexually active: 36 percent of 15- to 17-year-olds with romantic relationship experience have had sexual contact, compared with 12 percent of 13- to 14-year-olds with relationship experience.
- Teen pregnancy rates have steadily declined in the last few decades. Most recent data is around 16 births per

1,000 women ages 15 to 19. (For comparison, there were about 160 births per 1,000 women in their 20s, and around 150 births per 1,000 women in their 30s.)

▷ Around 54 percent of sexually active teens used a condom in their last sexual experience; 23 percent used birth control pills; 5 percent used an IUD or implant; 3 percent used a shot, patch, or ring; 10 percent used the with-drawal method; and 11 percent did not use any method to prevent pregnancy.

▷ One in four sexually active teens contracts a sexually transmitted infection (STI) each year. Estimates suggest that young people ages 15 to 24 consistently acquire half of all new STIs.

Sharing these kinds of stats with your son can prove to him that he has the power to choose for himself. No matter what he might think, not everyone is doing it—whatever "it" may be.

Example

Rohni (he/him) is 18. He has been sexually active for around 9 to 10 months. In that time, Rohni has, according to him, officially dated just one person. They were sexually active, and even though they broke up a few months ago, he considers it a nice relationship and a good learning experience. They still talk and hang out from time to time. On some occasions they still have sex. Love is out of the equation; the intimate part of the relationship is now purely and consensually physical. When they were dating, the relationship was exclusive, but since their breakup, Rohni has hooked up with two other people. He wouldn't consider them one-night stands, but Rohni doesn't know those partners very well and definitely doesn't know their sexual history. Rohni has used a condom in most, but not all, sexual contact.

Practical Guidelines

In Rohni's scenario, if his caregivers were knowledgeable about his sexual habits, they might focus their concern on safety and emotional intimacy. Rohni might benefit from some frank discussions about how consistent contraceptive efforts—and perhaps fewer sexual partners—would lower his risk. STI/HIV testing should also be a potential point of discussion, as well as a wellness check into his self-esteem. Rohni is considered an adult at his age, but his caregivers would be wise to consider if Rohni's sexual behavior is concerning to the point of intervention. But if they've successfully developed a relationship of trust, openness, and vulnerability with him, they should be able to assess if he's emotionally happy and healthy with his relationships.

Let's revisit three objectives from earlier in our chapters together to provide specific recommendations on safe sex and related conversations with your adolescent son.

Use correct terminology. Not all teenage relationships include sex, but by the numbers, many teenagers will experiment with sexual behavior at some stage. Therefore, you and your son need terminology and clear information on sexual contact, contraception, and sexually transmitted infections (STIs). STIs are preventable, but they are also treatable. Messages about safe sex should also eliminate stigma and present the truth: STIs don't mean someone is dirty or disgusting, but STIs are potentially dangerous, especially untreated.

Remain body- and sex-positive. This might be a tough truth to accept: Adolescents have the potential to become sexually active no matter the parental influence. Teens can find ways to engage in sexual contact despite our warnings and wishes. If we truly want our sons to be sexually safe, what seems more appropriate: exiling them to the backseat of a car parked in some remote area without access to birth control, or allowing discrete use of the rooms within his own household? This isn't condoning unhealthy underage sexual activity, but it is modeling care and positivity. You always have the ability to discuss appropriate and allowable behavior; your home, your rules. Yet opening said home and rules to be inclusive of the developing body and brain of your son might be the safest decision you can jointly make. Rohni's parents, though sex-positive in their discussions with their son, may have subtly signaled their discomfort with him bringing partners to their house. Coming to terms with reality will give them more opportunity to offer guidance and share the concerns they have.

Model lifelong learning. Your own beliefs about sex and virginity are unique and have a place in conversations with your son. So does modeling the willingness to continue to learn by hearing his side of the story and trying to understand what it's like for adolescents in today's world.

Open a Dialogue

Here are some examples of language use with your son regarding intimate moments and/or sexual contact. The goal is to offer a lasting, supportive message, so he can do what's best for himself. Notice the small plug for verbal confirmation at the end of each statement.

Abstinence

"Remember what we talked about. If there's drinking going on tonight, please be smart. That scares me. You know that. It also might lower your inhibitions. If you're not ready for sex, you don't have to do anything you don't want to do. Same for anyone else. Right?"

Contraception

"Hey bud. Just so you know, if you ever need birth control, just go ahead and pick some up from the store. If for any reason you can't, there are condoms in the hallway bathroom. This isn't a 'No questions asked' type of thing, but I just want you to be safe. Please use them whenever. Deal?"

Emergencies

"If you feel unsafe or threatened, I'm just a text or phone call away. You can always blame me. Say, 'My dad wants me home immediately. I gotta go.' I'll pay for a ride service, I'll come pick you up. Whatever it takes. Just get out of there if there's an emergency, okay?"

TAKEAWAYS

- Messages about safe sex shouldn't undermine sex positivity. The two go hand in hand; safe sex is pleasurable sex.
- Teens may find ways to be sexually active no matter their parents' wishes. As a caregiver you should make sure your son will be prepared and informed to stay safe.
- In dialogues with your son about safe sex, use proper terminology, remain body- and sex-positive, and model lifelong learning.

CHAPTER TWELVE

Challenging the Expectations of the Internet and Porn

In this chapter we will focus on an extremely sensitive, controversial subject: pornography. Whatever your opinion may be, the reality is that pornography is rampant online, and not just on websites that host pornographic content. The algorithms that influence and track your son's internet use will send porn his way in the form of social media videos, gifs and jpegs, static images, advertisements, and even the written word (think fan fiction). He doesn't have to seek out porn; it will find him.

The good news is that your hard work in all other facets of parenting through puberty will pay dividends in your conversations with him about pornography. Those countless talks and moments of connection establishing values, trust, and openness can help you ease into this tough topic with him. Add small moments of guidance here and there so he can become an educated internet user.

Background and Considerations

Pornography is the depiction of explicit sexual activity intended to cause sexual excitement. There are age restrictions across the world on pornography access; many areas require the adult age of 18. Because of the sensitivity of the topic, statistical information on pornography can vary, depending on the bias of whoever's doing the research. The dearth of valid statistics on pornography only reinforces the taboo and secretive nature of the subject, which is often part of the appeal, especially to young people.

Here's some credible data available at the time of publication:

- Nearly 70 percent of adolescents report having come across online pornography.
- About 42 percent of adolescents ages 10 to 17 were exposed to internet pornography in the past 12 months. An estimated 66 percent of those exposures were reported as unwanted.
- Some estimates put 4 to 5 percent of all websites as carrying pornography, with as high as 15 percent of internet searches relating to porn.

Before discussing the subject with your son in earnest, it's important that you have a clear understanding of your own views about porn. Once you feel ready to open the dialogue, consider the following points and potential negative impact when bringing the subject of pornography into your parent-son conversations.

Not discussing pornography at all. You're already invested in your son's adolescent development. Pornography is just another essential discussion point on the list of sexual wellness topics. Teens categorically explain that most of the "sex education" they get is from pornography. Even with a quality sex ed program in school, your son needs you to offer perspective. And avoiding the topic will not make it go away.

Thinking he won't be exposed to it. Pop-up advertisements, incorrect search results, and misleading website titles can yield pornographic content, not to mention his peers, who may share pictures and videos. Even with all internet filters and parental controls operating perfectly, the only way to completely block your son from accessing porn, purposely *or* accidentally, is to keep him offline indefinitely. This is quite implausible.

Believing that discussing porn is an endorsement or condemnation. Your conversations about pornography do not mean you are for or against it. As we've established, porn exists. So having a sex-positive talk about porn doesn't mean you support your son accessing it. And creating a dialogue about porn's harmful messages doesn't suggest you believe all who use it are immoral. You are merely working on porn literacy together.

Presuming that talking about porn creates an interest in it. This is simply not statistically accurate. As with drug use, suicide, and sex, educating your teen about the topic will not cause him to become more interested in it than he already was.

Not recognizing a problem. Signs that pornography has become a problem in your son's life include: hidden phone use, quickly logging off when you're around, loss of interest in previous hobbies, sudden and uncharacteristic drop in grades, sleep struggles, sexual language, excessive masturbation, and defensiveness about internet use. If you're concerned, check his browsing history and/or ask your son outright: "Can I see what you've been up to online?"

Jalen (he/him) is 12 years old. While hanging out in his friend's bedroom, they say to him, "You've got to see this video I saw on the internet. It's crazy." It's a pornographic internet site and related message board. Jalen's parents have specifically spoken with him about porn; their discussions were sex-positive but full of legitimate warnings about the intense imagery and potential messages Jalen might want to stay away from at his age. Jalen's family has always had family settings on their media devices; Jalen recently got his own phone and agreed to fair guidelines for using it. His parents have done their best to build a trust in Jalen to do what's right for himself, but they knew through neighborhood friends that there was some recent porn exposure and website sharing going on among some of the boys in the community. Before he knows it, Jalen's friend is playing the video, and it is indeed explicit sex acts from adults on a porn website.

Practical Guidelines

Jalen's scenario is a common one. His caregivers have seemingly done a solid job of preempting his porn use as a preteen, but there are always other avenues to exposure. Internet settings may block some sexual content, but substantive conversations with your son are a better remedy. The objective is to help your son analyze what media he chooses to consume and assess how to handle what isn't his choice. Here are some lines of reasoning and words of advice to use in these conversations:

Entertainment is not reality. Almost all porn is a work of fiction. Pornography is scripted sex strictly for its own sake. As an adult, you know this, but you'll want your son to internalize this fact, too. Pornography is not going to help a curious teen learn how to act or what do to in a real-world sexual relationship. And a teenager is absolutely able to comprehend that.

It's okay to say "no." Despite public perception, not every teenage boy watches porn. In some ways, talking about how to handle the pressure to view porn is like talking about going to a party. As you and your son discuss potential refusal skills, let him know he can always lean on values and household rules. Jalen can turn away with a simple, "I'm not allowed, no thanks." If your son's friends pressure him with porn constantly, it'll be time for a decision. Are these really friends he wants to be around?

Declare what you don't do instead of what you can't do. This is a common refusal skill for underage drinking or other risky behaviors. If Jalen says, "I can't," it can sound like it's just this one time, or he needs convincing. If he says, "I don't do that," he gets straight to the truth. This has a direct application to consent as well. He is opting not to, as a conscious decision, and a true friend will respect that.

Open a Dialogue

Your son might not believe that his online activity is risky or harmful. You can create appropriate concern regarding porn's impact on his psyche by appealing to his freedom of choice. These ideas are especially useful for an older teen.

Him: *"It's not that big a deal."*

You: *"That might be true. And that's okay to believe if you are feeling unaffected by pornography. But it's also alright for something to matter. This matters to me. As do you. That's why it's necessary to know the difference between porn as entertainment and sexual contact as real intimacy. Can we talk about it further?"*

Him: *"I hardly watch any."*

You: *"That's fine. And you're not in trouble. You can navigate your own way around the internet, and I want you to be able to do so. But it's the same as practicing safe, consensual sex: It's important for porn to bring pleasure without harm to anyone involved, you included. Do you have any questions about what you see?"*

Him: *"You just don't understand."*

You: *"No, I don't. I have no idea what it's truly like to be a teenager in this day and age. But I do understand that the choices you make today need to be the choices you can live with tomorrow. I care about you, that's all. Can you help me understand a little more about your feelings on things?"*

TAKEAWAYS

▶ Opinions on pornography vary, and unbiased statistics are hard to come by.

▶ Whatever your opinion on porn, there's no question that your son will be exposed to it online, even if he doesn't seek it out. Ignoring the issue won't make it go away, and talking about it won't make him interested in it.

▶ Your son should understand that pornography is acting, that no one should pressure him to watch it, and that his online activity can always be traced.

CHAPTER THIRTEEN

Discussing Texting and Social Media

Staying safe in today's digital era means understanding that not everything needs to be shared, and not everything needs to be consumed. Like it or not, social media platforms are part of modern life; indeed, our teens never knew a world without them. Texting, messaging, and scrolling are as much a part of teenage life today as were renting videos, making mixtapes, and hanging out at the mall for a previous generation. What's important is that your son knows how to use these tools in safe, benign, and appropriate ways, and what to do when things go wrong. In this chapter we'll explore the best practices for raising a savvy user of social media.

Background and Considerations

A relationship can manifest online through social media or texting, but if there is never face-to-face human interaction, the typical connection for a healthy relationship is bypassed. This isn't to say that exclusively online relationships can't work, but they are more difficult to pull off. It's hard to develop the depth of intimacy needed for a lasting, successful relationship when there's no in-person physical closeness.

Many teenagers say texting and social media are the best options to flirt with a crush or romantic interest, even ahead of in-person interaction. Most teenage romantic relationships do not start online, but that statistic could be in an upswing, with more platforms and apps popping up each year aimed specifically at teenagers.

Just how ubiquitous are these things for today's teenagers? At the time of publication:

- Up to 95 percent of teens have access to a smartphone, and 45 percent say they are online "almost constantly."
- About 31 percent of teens say social media has had a mostly positive impact, whereas 24 percent describe its effect as mostly negative.
- Around 50 percent of teens have let someone know they were interested in them romantically by connecting with them on social media ("friending" or "following").
- Approximately 47 percent of teens have expressed their attraction by liking, commenting, or otherwise interacting with that person on social media.
- Roughly 55 percent of teens ages 13 to 17 have flirted with or talked to someone in person to let them know they are interested.

- Roughly 46 percent of teens have shared something funny or interesting with their romantic interest online.
- About 10 percent of teens have sent flirtatious or sexy pictures or videos of themselves.
- Between 5 to 7 percent of teens have made a sexually revealing video for a partner or potential partner.

Demands for sexual texts, or threats of spreading any shared nude photos, are illegal in many areas and are additional warning signs of toxic, abusive relationships. You've probably heard the term "sexting," which refers to the sending of nude or sexually suggestive images electronically, whether through text messaging, social media, chat boards, or email. It is important to know that sexting laws vary tremendously across nations and across the states. Teenage sexting can lead to felony charges and appearance on sex offender lists, since nude photos or videos of someone under the age of 18 could be considered child pornography. These serious consequences make it worth your while to research your community's statutes and review them with your son.

Example

Phillip (he/him) is 18 years old. He is angry he can't get the attention of his ex-girlfriend after their breakup. In the middle of the night, at 3:00 a.m., Phillip forwards some sexually explicit images of his ex as a means of getting a reaction. She had consensually texted them to Phillip while they were together, but she was 16 at the time. Phillip not only sends the photos to friends, but he also texts them to her friends and her family. Phillip is arrested for distributing explicit photos of a minor, constituting child pornography. He is tried in court and required to register as a sex offender.

Practical Guidelines

You can see that things can escalate and quickly become out of control for a socially-emotionally immature teen who has access to an internet device or is around others who do.

Undoubtedly, as a caregiver you want some recommendations for aiding your son's online behavior. You also want to know how he can remain safe, appropriate, and legal with his habits. And you will want to help him enjoy social media without falling into the negative aspects of the internet community. Let's dive into the specifics.

Start early. As with conversations about healthy relationships, consent, and safe sex, caregivers can nurture life skills regarding social media early on. Behaviors like sexting may show up earlier than caregivers expect, so it's best to stay ahead with early discussions in terms that your son can understand. Explicit mention of sexual imagery is not necessary to get the point across; simply explain how your values, like courtesy, respect, and privacy, apply to online communications.

Keep your head about texting and sexting. Let's clarify a truth regarding sexting: Exchanging flirtatious or sexy texts, pictures, or videos can be part of a healthy relationship. Emphasis on the word *can*. In adulthood, we have the necessary inhibitory responses ingrained into the decision-making portions of the brain that help keep us safe from potential harm. Consenting adults can use sexting either as a form of foreplay or to strengthen intimacy. But teenagers often mimic this behavior without the reward of a closer connection to their partner. And without the trust of privacy.

If you find sexting or nude photos have been spread by your son, there are definitely concerns about legality. It's normal for parents to feel scared or ashamed or embarrassed, but never, ever cover things up. Model honesty and owning up to mistakes in life. In Phillip's scenario, caregivers need to contact any other parents as necessary and cooperate with authorities or school administration if it comes to that.

Discuss social media practices. When your son enters the social media sphere—depending on your family rules—emphasize media as an extension of oneself. Humor, music, sports, arts, dance, tech, and even harmless memes are all appropriate ways to post to friends and followers.

Bullying and harassing, in contrast, are not an appropriate, constructive use of social media. Most boys understand that this behavior isn't acceptable in person, so it shouldn't be part of their online behavior, either. Would Phillip have exposed his ex that way if he'd had to look everyone in the eye as he distributed the images? Does he really want people he meets to think of him as a person who would do that? Probably not.

Most media experts recommend waiting until at least age 13 for social media. It's also okay for adolescents to stay off media apps or gaming platforms completely. You and your family should decide against it until the right time. In order to keep tabs on things, ask to be connected or require access to your son's social media accounts; that's certainly fair until he turns 17 or 18. Encourage him to see social media as an extension of his social life, not a replacement. Real-life relationships and activities build the brain in ways that a screen cannot. Also remind him that pictures in the digital realm cannot be truly erased, so think twice before posting online or sending a picture to someone.

Open a Dialogue

Drawing awareness to internet safety and appropriate online behavior doesn't have to be complicated. Start with the basics from the acronym THINK, which represents questions that your son—or anyone—should quickly go through before posting something.

T: Is this true?

Is what you are sharing factual? Or is it just an opinion or emotion? Knowing this can help with clarity on your message.

H: Is this helpful?

Does your message help you or others, or does it assist with a certain situation?

I: Is this inspiring?

Have you thought about how your message might affect someone's mood?

N: Is this necessary?

Would your messages be better left unsent? Could you speak to someone face-to-face instead?

K: Is this kind?

What's your motivation for sharing this message?

TAKEAWAYS

- Social media and texting are embedded in modern life. Our teens need to learn to use them safely and appropriately.
- It's okay for online communication to be part of a relationship, but it can't be a substitute for in-person contact.
- Your son can learn to apply routine thinking before he posts or texts: Is this message true, helpful, inspiring, necessary, and kind?

CHAPTER FOURTEEN

Raising an Ally

Our final chapter focus is on enabling one of the most precious gifts in your life to pay it forward and share his best qualities with others. Child-rearing takes patience and persistence, and, over time, it takes letting go of control and moving into cooperation. Because he's witnessed this behavior in you, your son can exhibit this behavior in himself, such as providing support, assistance, and service to others. This is what it means to be an ally, or—in other words—a kind and contributing human being. Our final chapter will help you point the way for your son to follow this positive, altruistic path through adolescence and into adulthood.

Background and Considerations

Orienting your son to be an ally amplifies the values that you've taught him to affect others in the community for the better. Being an ally, or allyship, is the practice of emphasizing social justice, inclusion, and human rights. More specifically, an ally advances the interests of typically oppressed or marginalized individuals or mistreated groups. An ally supports other people, plain and simple, through words and action. It's not just hope for a better future; it means actively doing something to create that future through solidarity. It's compassion and empathy put into practice.

Advocacy is public support or recommendation of a particular cause, idea, or policy. Advocacy is a piece of being an ally. It puts support into action. Being an ally is also recognizing the advantages, opportunities, resources, and influence one automatically has in life. And like any alliance, everyone benefits.

As your son takes a wider interest in the world around him, and you begin having conversations about values and openness, these topics are important jumping off points to begin your discussions.

Wealth disparity. The wealth gap in modern society is far and wide. In the United States, the richest top 5 percent of families hold over 200 times as much wealth as the median income.

Discrimination and violence against women. About one out of every six women has been the victim of an attempted or completed rape in her lifetime. Up to 90 percent of all sexual assault victims are women. In the gender pay gap, women earn around 84 percent what men earn annually.

Discrimination and violence against LGBTQ (Lesbian, Gay, Bisexual, Transgender, Queer) individuals. Discrimination is common for LGBTQ adults, with 57 percent reporting experiencing slurs, 51 percent reporting sexual harassment, 51 percent reporting violence, and 34 percent reporting harassment regarding restroom use.

Discrimination and violence against Black people, Indigenous People, and people of color. Racial disparities exist in arrests and incarceration rates for Black and Indigenous individuals. The wealth discrepancy is equally as wide. Median Black household income is around 60 percent of median white household income.

Discrimination and violence against people with disabilities. Students with disabilities—physical, developmental, and emotional—face more challenges both academicaly and socially. These challenges don't stop once they're out of school. An estimated 82 percent of people who have disabilities live below the poverty line.

Issues facing the elderly. About 82 percent of seniors report experiencing stereotypes, prejudice, or discrimination based on their age.

Example

Remember our example with Ry from chapter six? Here are some further details from later in Ry's life story.

High schooler Ry (they/them) is using social media platforms to show solidarity with causes that are close to their heart—Ry is especially committed to sharing racial justice and body-positive messages. Ry's friends were highly concerned with their school's lack of access to menstrual products in the restrooms. Even though it didn't directly impact Ry, they helped create a pitch for the school board to approve. Funding was successfully obtained for restroom dispensers and supplies. Ry is also a part of the peer buddy program that partners nondisabled students with students with disabilities. Ry's parents are proud, but also worry that these activities will take time away from their academics.

Practical Guidelines

Here are some considerations for fostering your son's burgeoning allyship.

Be supportive. If you have any concerns about your son's activities, remain wholehearted, authentic, and a role model for kindness when you express them. Be honest about your feelings in regard to your son's beliefs and actions. If the causes he supports don't match your own choices, could it be that you need updated facts? Young people are often on the pulse of world affairs; your son may be able to turn the tables and help educate you. If his advocacy seems to be misdirected, work on influencing him toward a different direction, not controlling him. Whatever the case, remember that he is still learning.

Help them make wider connections. If a particular cause seems to be truly close to your son's heart, discuss ways that he might plan involvement over the long term. He may feel less pressured to spend every free moment on it and begin to pace himself more realistically. In Ry's case, their interest in helping people with special needs has them considering a college career program in the field. This means Ry needs to keep up with their schoolwork as well as volunteering.

Champion positive masculinity. Whereas toxic masculinity might focus on bodies in terms of pride and celebration, as if sex is a conquest delineating a boy's virile transition into manhood, positive masculinity focuses on the human body as a tool for personal, relational, and societal betterment. Draw your son's attention to the amount of sexism, and sex in general, that he may be exposed to online. Your son and his peers have an influence on where social media is heading and direct control on how texting fits into social health.

Encourage purpose. The teen years can help establish the foundation for deeper connections in committed, fulfilling, adult relationships. One important way for your son to build a life of allyship and advocacy is to develop purpose. Purpose is aim and intention in life. It is the reason for action and the determination to achieve and "become." Remind your son that he is creating his future, one day at a time. Being an ally and advocate gives boys the awareness that they have something worthwhile to say and contribute.

Open a Dialogue

Here are some discussion points you can raise when helping your son find his footing as he develops his practice as an ally:

If you're concerned he's spreading himself too thin . . .

"I admire the work you're doing, but you won't be able to help if you burn yourself out, right? How can you approach this cause as a marathon, not a sprint?"

If you have doubts about the direction he's taking . . .

"I'm not sure I have all the facts about this advocacy group you're involved with. Can you tell me more about it, and can I ask some questions?"

If he seems hesitant to become an involved citizen . . .

"I know that some kids your age do volunteer work and some don't, and either is okay with me. Just helping and sticking up

for people in your everyday life is important, too. But remember that volunteering is a good way to meet new people, and it can help with college admissions, too. If there's ever a cause you might want to get involved with in some minor way, I'd be happy to help you explore the options."

TAKEAWAYS

▸ An ally supports other people through words and actions. It's a natural progression for an adolescent boy who's been raised to appreciate trust, respect, openness, vulnerability, and the values you've imparted to him.

▸ Our sons can play an important role in propagating positive masculinity and an antidote to toxic masculinity.

▸ Allyship benefits our sons by giving them purpose. As caregivers, we can help our sons become allies without overcommitting themselves or risking their own well-being.

PART IV

FREQUENTLY ASKED QUESTIONS, ANSWERED

Your work to build a bond leading up to this point in your son's life matters. All of those efforts have a positive influence on how things will go for the remainder of his teen years. The hope is this book has served as a jumping-off point for having courageous conversations about relationships and sex. The general ideas combined with specific scenarios were meant to get the wheels turning for your own parent-son interactions.

Through it all, recall our basic objectives for your parenting journey: Aim for correct terminology, stay body-positive, and remain open to lifelong learning. You care, and it shows. To help you further, I've compiled 25 questions that seem to come up time and again.

1. *How do I know when my son is starting puberty?*

Answer: Signs of physical development are constant through adolescence—from height and weight gain to changing facial features—but the first noticeable signs of puberty will be different for every child. Secondary sex characteristics, as they're called, include a deepening voice, acne, an increase in body hair, muscle development, and even early mood swings. Be on the lookout for any and all to be showing up anywhere from ages 9 to 14 and continue until ages 16 to 19.

2. *What should be my first conversation topic about puberty or relationships? What's the biggest issue he may need help with?*

Answer: Naturally, pressing issues depend on the child. You don't need a "first" conversation topic, because as a caregiver, you're always talking about life. Educating a young person about the world is the beginning of your dialogues about puberty. Undoubtedly, you've already helped with topics of growth and development by discussing how the body works, why we stay clean with hygiene, and eating and exercise habits. If you haven't covered "where babies come from," do so as soon as possible. Use simple, accurate information. This can be done in small conversations with short bursts of information, especially at bedtime when the daily routine feels less rushed.

3. *What's the best way to help him feel comfortable coming to me with questions?*

Answer: Tone and body language can go along with the consistent message that you care. But be more specific than just, *"I'm here if you need anything."* Boys may not reach out of their own accord. Ask simple questions about his day, just like any conversation, and plug in things you notice. Has he grown recently? Ask about underwear needs. Does he need a razor and shaving kit? Ask him to go with you to pick something out. Is he starting to date? Find out his thoughts on attraction and intimacy. Depending on his age, ask about everything from deodorant to social media, from emotions to contraception needs. Be up-front! *"Do you need any condoms?"* may be weird at first, but for an older teen especially, it puts the notion in his head that you are open to saying the words and therefore open to receiving questions about sex. If he gets embarrassed that it's too awkward, restate the constant truth: You just want to help him stay safe, healthy, and happy.

4. *I am noticing a need for cleanliness and deodorant. Frankly, he's starting to smell. How can I help my son with better hygiene?*

Answer: Buy him deodorant! Enforce strict shower habits by making it the same time every day. After the shower, observe that he's including deodorant along with dental care, hair care, and other bodily maintenance. If he is physically active, have him shower and change clothes afterward as well. Get him good clothing and even a change of underwear for physical education class, plus extra deodorant for school.

5. *My son needs help with manners and consideration for others. He's very immature. What can I do to help his maturity level?*

Answer: Draw attention on the spot to anything that seems selfish, without making a scene. Be firm while remaining careful of your tone, as he'll respond to appeals to his social health instead of yelling rants. *"When you do that, it can make others feel _____."* Use outside examples to create metaphors for his own behavior. As annoying as it may be, you'll need to offer nearly constant reminders on table manners, bodily functions, and being polite when speaking. This is the thankless work of parenting a preteen in particular. Call him out on unsavory behavior and make sure to point out the positives, even small items, when he does something considerate.

6. *When do I bring up the topic of sex? What's the right age?*

Answer: There isn't a right or wrong age for discussing sexual wellness since this depends on his development and interest. Start conversations early in childhood for continuity through teen years. If you haven't started, it isn't too late—get going right away with age-appropriate topics. Is he young? Begin with bodies and babies. Is he a preteen? Work through expected puberty changes and relationship development. Is he a teen? Stay consistent on dating, intimacy, and internet use (texting, social media, pornography).

7. *How can I bridge the topic of masturbation without making it weird?*

Answer: A calm tone and straightforward wording are important when discussing self-pleasure. Avoid shame, as always. If he feels any guilt on his own, affirm that self-touch is pleasurable and normal to explore. If the question is about appropriate timing or number of weekly occurrences, establish boundaries just like any activity—video games, snack foods, etc. There is a time and place where masturbation fits into growing up, but it needs to mesh with privacy needs and other life activities. Share any values you need to discuss about pornography in the meantime.

8. *I don't want to seem too involved or pushy, but how can I get my son birth control access?*

Answer: If you have the relationship comfort to research things together, particularly with an older teen, do so with guidance from your primary care physician. Start off with help as needed, but ensure it isn't just you doing the legwork to get products for protection or contraception. He needs to learn how to access and use it on his own for independence in sexual wellness. If he finds your involvement too awkward, stay persistent. Deep down it is registering that you care; any awkwardness will diminish with time.

9. *What if I walk in on my son with a partner during sexual contact?*

Answer: If you walk in on him, or even if he walks in on you, don't worry that he'll be scarred for life. Sex is not shameful. You can use it as a teachable moment about privacy, or, if a simple mistake was made, make an apology and move forward. Teens often explain that although having a supportive caregiver can play a positive role in their life, not everything needs a lesson. Check that he's being safe and the intimacy is consensual, and that might be it. If he is a preteen and you're worried about his young age, seek out a counselor for the appropriate course of action. If he's older, perhaps this allows you to plan respectful, noninvasive signals about vicinity and privacy (lights on/off, knocking, or noise up/downstairs, etc.).

10. *I believe my son is questioning his sexuality and/or his gender identity. I know he may identify as part of the LGBTQ community, but I'm not sure he wants to come out yet. Is there anything I can or should be doing?*

Answer: Behaving positively and nonjudgmentally is a good first step. A big part of this is being clear about your own feelings about sexuality and gender identity. You can help with sex-positive resources (check the Resources section or scour your local library) or with simple, affirming comments during movies or TV shows with representation, but do not try to force things. Sexuality is not everyone's business. If he wants to come out to you, he will. If not, allow him space to grow and figure out what he wants in life. If you think your child is questioning their gender, be positive and loving, and offer them resources. Whatever you do, don't react by enforcing gender norms upon them. PFLAG is a great resource for parents of queer and trans kids.

11. *My son is an older teen, and I think he is nervous about dating. He seems to believe everyone else is in relationships and may be having sex. I don't think he's ready, but he's definitely feeling the pressure from his social circle. How can I help his mindset that "everyone is doing it"?*

Answer: Start with this simple fact: Relationships and sexual contact are not linked to self-worth. Intimacy and sexuality are unique for everyone. Having frequent or infrequent partners or sexual contact is not connected to desirability or life satisfaction. He has plenty of time to figure out his needs and desires! Even if he's in a relationship, encourage your son to drop self-judgment surrounding sex. Chances are that he knows not everyone is in a relationship; perhaps it's just a few close friends and he's feeling left out. A plug here or there to branch out to new friends is plenty: *"Maybe there are some other people who aren't dating you can reach out to. We're heading over to _____ as a family—you're welcome to ask them to join if you like."*

12. *I think my son has been watching porn. What should I do?*

Answer: First, try not to panic or shame. Your son is either looking for education or entertainment. What values about bodies, relationships, and sex have you already communicated with him? What do you want him to gain from your conversation(s)? Establishing boundaries may be needed. However, stating, *"Not in this household!"* doesn't ensure he won't view porn outside of the home and doesn't hit the main theme here—education about the potential imagery and messages he is consuming. Focus on the intent of porn as entertainment and not reality—that it may have a place in sexuality and relationships, but excessive exposure can harm his view on gender roles and real-life situations.

13. *How can I help my son navigate time on social media and the internet? He is online almost constantly. I wish he'd look up from his phone.*

Answer: Even though your relationship with your son is a mutual, collaborative effort, remember you have the final call. You're the parent, so set up expectations on screen time, even if you don't have any yet. Monitor time with built-in apps. Expect pushback but assure your son that you're not trying to take his phone away—that won't happen unless he makes a major mistake online. Come to an agreement on how many posts he can make a week and perhaps how many direct messages he can send and receive. Other ideas: phones down during dinner; phones away when company visits; phones off until homework is done; and, above all else, eye contact and full attention when speaking with someone. Be prepared to model behavior with devices by adhering to family guidelines yourself. Stay consistent and firm without arguing and see if in-person communication improves.

14. *I don't want to stifle my son's natural inclination to be male. Masculinity can be a good thing, right? Can you further explain positive masculinity?*

Answer: We absolutely want young males to be proud of their bodies and life potential. As an example, athleticism has an important place in the history of men, with many aspects to celebrate—the competitive challenge, the personal betterment, the camaraderie with fellow athletes, the discipline in training, and the ability to help others. Other progressive manly attributes could include moral courage, involved fatherhood, and advocating for others. With our help, masculinity can continue to be constructive, not destructive, as boys learn to build themselves up without tearing others down.

15. *Are there any quick tips I should share for effective condom use?*

Answer: Always refer to a reputable source like the WHO or CDC. Condoms are anywhere from 85 to 98 percent effective, but that ranges because of user error. Correct use: (1) Carefully unwrap the condom and place it on the head of the erect penis. If intact, pull back the foreskin first. (2) Pinch air out of the tip of the condom. (3) Unroll the condom all the way down the penis. (4) After sexual activity, hold the condom at the base of the penis until away from partner. (5) Be mindful with a used condom—tie it off or wrap it in toilet paper, then place it in the garbage instead of the toilet. Never leave it out.

16. *What are all the options and effectiveness I can pass on to my son for contraception and STI prevention?*

Answer:
For contraception:

External condom = latex, plastic, or lambskin sheath that covers the penis or other object before sex. One time use (85 percent effective).

Internal condom = soft plastic pouch inserted into vagina or anus before sex. One time use (79 percent effective).

Withdrawal method = "pulling out" to ejaculate away from the vulva (78 percent effective).

Abstinence = not engaging in sexual contact (100 percent effective, when observed). Effective protection against STIs.

Birth control pill = daily medication. Releases hormones to block ovulation/fertilization (91 percent effective).

Intrauterine device (IUD) = placed into uterus by health-care provider. Releases hormones to block fertilization. Lasts up to 10 years (99 percent effective).

Implant = thin rod placed in upper arm by health-care provider. Releases hormones to block fertilization. Lasts up to five years (99 percent effective).

Emergency contraception = "morning after" IUD or pill used up to five days after unprotected sex. Releases hormones to block fertilization (75 to 89 percent effective).

Others = shot, patch, ring, sponge, diaphragm, cervical cap, barriers/dental dams, fertility awareness/rhythm method.

For STIs:

External condom = latex, plastic, or lambskin sheath that covers the penis or other object before sex. One time use (85 percent effective).

Internal condom = soft plastic pouch inserted into vagina or anus before sex. One time use (79 percent effective).

Gardasil = for HPV (Human papillomavirus).

Truvada and Descovy = PrEP (pre-exposure prophylaxes), which can prevent people who are at risk from getting HIV.

17. *My son has a disability. As he ages, I want to provide the right information on puberty and sexual wellness, but I need it to match his level of understanding/ability. Any help?*

Answer: As many as 1 in 10 people around the world lives with a disability. Like everyone else, people with disabilities must manage stigma—individuals with disabilities are sexual, too. His school might have ideas on appropriate books or lessons on puberty growth. Lean on those experts who have previously worked through the topics with other kids. Maintain boundaries of helping versus enabling during hygiene routines (have him do as much on his own as he is physically or mentally able), and discuss safe sex with the same matter-of-fact description as other behaviors (eating, exercise, screen time). Keep an eye out for resources specific to his developmental disorder or disability; there are often social media groups where parents can find each other for ideas and support.

18. *My son just went through a breakup. They were close for quite a while, and the whole family got to know his dating partner well, so we're all a bit sad, actually. What can I do to help?*

Answer: It is natural for you as the parent to feel sadness and loss yourself after your son goes through a breakup, particularly if you have all spent a lot of time together. You've developed your own emotional intimacy, and, although on a different level than your son, you're allowed to experience grief as well. More important, support your son's emotional well-being. Help him see a future without his ex. Encourage him to stay active in other activities and remain off social media, and relay the consistent message that any feelings of regret or longing will dissipate over time.

19. *My son doesn't seem to care too strongly about much. He just doesn't see a point in following world events. I am hoping to help him work on his empathy and allyship capabilities. How can I get him to be a helpful, considerate, contributing person without pushing too hard or in the wrong way?*

Answer: First, know that it's not just your child. Motivation to do *anything* can be a struggle with teens—to do homework, tidy their room, wear presentable clothes . . . you name it. Although it's frustrating as a parent, remember that they're still learning. This might be the time to model your own involvement and solidarity with others, drawing attention to how the world is interrelated and benefits from collective contributions. Continue to talk about timely examples of allyship you see in current events or in fiction. Still nothing? You can try showing him the real-life consequences if you stop doing certain things for/with him compared to working together. Tough love might work, or it might not. Always praise the times he does get involved, so positive feedback can slowly shift his mindset.

20. *My son makes inappropriate jokes. I've also caught wind that he posts some questionable stuff on his social media page from time to time as well. I'm worried he's growing up to be inconsiderate and flat-out mean. What can I do?*

Answer: Disrespect is an area where a major parenting decision needs to be made. Whether it's inappropriate posts and comments, knowingly mean behavior, or full-out bullying, you'll want to nip the issue in the bud. What's the consequence? Online access will need monitoring, but you may have to temporarily take away internet or phone privileges. Obviously, he can find other ways to get online; for that reason behavioral change through positive discussions and education is the goal. But if you're beyond that, reel him back in and *then* have quality conversations during and after a short "probationary period" off devices. A screenless weekend will feel like eternity to him. In the meantime, can you get to the root of the behavior? Ultimately, if things are severe, you may need to seek help from a professional to see if there are any underlying issues.

21. *One of my son's friends came out as transgender. They've been friends since childhood, and I've gotten to know this other person well over the years. I got the new name down, but I just can't seem to get their new pronouns right. I feel horrible about it. I really want to do the right thing, and I'm not trying to be disrespectful, so how can I break the old pronoun habit?*

Answer: This is a valid concern and by asking such a question, you obviously care. The basic answer is best here: Stick with it. Over time, your interactions with them in their transition will reestablish pronouns in your brain. And practice their pronouns when they are not around. If you make a mistake, quickly apologize and make the correction. Stating the obvious is respectful, too—*"I'm sorry I keep screwing up. I fully support you, but I know I keep using the wrong pronouns. I apologize for that. I've known you so long and my brain is still adjusting."*

22. *I'm concerned about my son's behavior toward women. I think he's been making sexual comments about girls and has a sexy picture as the background on his phone. He's always making comments to his friends like, "Will there be girls there? Hot ones?" What can I do to help?*

Answer: In this case, multiple conversations will be needed to combat growing toxic behavior and replace it with positive masculinity. Dating is not a conquest. Others do not solely exist for our pleasure. And even if he's getting reactions, especially from male friends, explain that the treatment of women in this regard is harmful and inappropriate. Stay steady in your demands for respect for other genders, with examples of women in your family as analogies, if needed. Would he want his mother/sister/grandmother being treated this way? If his words and actions are over the line of concern and consistently sexist, time for consequences—consider revoking privileges until he improves his behavior.

23. *I'm finding this "sex-positive" thing a little overwhelming. I mean, I don't want my son having sex, right? I want him waiting until way later in life. Don't I?*

Answer: That might be true. Your son might benefit from more committed relationships before sexual contact. And you can only approach things with the lens of your own past; prolonging sexual contact may have worked for you, or you may feel you engaged in sex too early. But every teen creates their own life, with their own choices. Do your best to leave an impact with multiple conversations about values, relationship attachment, and safe, protected sexual contact. In the end, however, your son needs to find a path into sexuality that works for him. Use care and love to support, support, support.

24. *I don't want to scare my son away from sex, but I do want to keep him away from sexually transmitted diseases and teen pregnancy. Is there a way to do that without scare tactics and without adding more stigma to STIs or pregnancy?*

Answer: Parents won't find much long-term success in scare tactics or presenting sex as scary. That said, wanting your teen to be safe with sexual contact is smart! Instead of terming pregnancy as this risky, horrible side effect of sexual contact, describe it as a wonderful and major life decision worthy of respect and admiration. This respect can help with timing of sexual contact. If he's in a heterosexual relationship, discuss with your son the commitment it takes to be a parent. With STIs, the truth matters once again. They are in fact treatable, but they can come with complications. If your son will be engaging in sexual contact no matter what, help him with access and options for protection and contraception (and how to correctly use them).

25. *Are there any random items that might go overlooked or unmentioned as someone is developing into a sexual person?*

Answer: Here are some final quotes—some blunt, some more profound—that may help get your gears turning with regard to a comprehensive look at puberty, relationships, and sexual wellness. All are informally worded, as though you are speaking directly to your son.

- "Consider your partner. Always. When in doubt, just ask."
- "It's okay if you are not interested in sex."
- "Lube goes a long way in helping comfort and pleasure."
- "In a new relationship, you won't know what works until you figure it out together."
- "Masturbation is always an option for safe sex."
- "There is no rush. You are worth waiting for."
- "Orgasms are not the only standard for sexual satisfaction."
- "Pee after sex. It may help prevent urinary tract infections (UTIs)."
- "There is more to intimacy than sex."

RESOURCES

Advocates For Youth. AdvocatesForYouth.org.

Amaze. Amaze.org.

Belge, Kathy and Marke Bieschke. *Queer: The Ultimate LGBTQ Guide for Teens*. Minneapolis: Lerner Publishing Group, 2019.

Brown, Brené. *Daring Greatly: How the Courage to Be Vulnerable Transforms the Way We Live, Love, Parent, and Lead*. London: Penguin, 2015.

Corinna, Heather and Isabella Rotman. *Wait, What?: A Comic Book Guide to Relationships, Bodies, and Growing Up*. Portland, OR: Limerence Press, 2019.

"Digital Citizenship Resource List." Harvard Graduate School of Education. October 2018. MCC.GSE.Harvard.edu /resources-for-educators/digital-citizenship-resource-list.

Dweck, Carol. *Mindset: The New Psychology of Success*. London: Robinson, 2017.

GLSEN. GLSEN.org.

Gonzales, Kathryn and Karen Rayne. *Trans+: Love, Sex, Romance, and Being You*. Washington: American Psychological Association, 2019.

Hazlett, Alex. "Here's Why Sex Ed Should Begin As Early As Possible." Parents.com. June 10, 2021. Parents.com/kids/development /heres-why-sex-ed-should-begin-as-early-as-possible.

I Wanna Know. IWannaKnow.org.

KidsHealth. *Nemours Foundation*. KidsHealth.org.

Loveless, Gina. *Puberty Is Gross but Also Really Awesome*. Toronto: Rodale Kids, 2021.

Natterson, Cara. *Guy Stuff: The Body Book for Boys*. Middleton, WI: American Girl Publishing, 2017.

"Male Reproductive System." *TeensHealth*. Nemours Foundation. September 2016. KidsHealth.org/en/teens/male-repro.html.

Mardell, Ashley. *The ABC's of LGBT+*. Miami: Mango Publishing, 2021.

PFLAG. PFLAG.org.

Rough, Bonnie J. *Beyond Birds & Bees: Bringing Home a New Message to Our Kids About Sex, Love, and Equality*. New York: Seal Press, 2018.

Scarleteen. Scarleteen.com.

Sex, Etc. SexEtc.org.

Sex Positive Families. SexPositiveFamilies.com.

Six Minute Sex Ed. TeaAndIntimacyCom.wordpress.com.

Stay Teen. StayTeen.org.

Taylor, Sonya Renee. *Celebrate Your Body (And Its Changes, Too!)* Emeryville, CA: Rockridge Press, 2018.

Todnem, Scott. *Growing Up Great! The Ultimate Puberty Book for Boys*. Emeryville, CA: Rockridge Press, 2019.

Vernacchio, Al. *For Goodness Sex: Changing the Way We Talk to Teens About Sexuality, Values, and Health*. New York: Harper Wave, 2014.

"What Consent Looks Like." *RAINN*. RAINN.org/articles /what-is-consent.

Youth Activism Project. YouthActivismProject.org.

Zaloom, Shafia. *Sex, Teens, & Everything in Between: The New and Necessary Conversations Today's Teenagers Need to Have about Consent, Sexual Harassment, Healthy Relationships, Love, and More*. Naperville, IL: Sourcebooks, 2019.

REFERENCES

"Adolescent Mental Health." World Health Organization. September 28, 2020. WHO.int/news-room/fact-sheets/detail /adolescent-mental-health.

"Adverse Childhood Experiences (ACEs)." Centers for Disease Control and Prevention. Last modified April 2, 2021. CDC.gov /violenceprevention/aces/index.html.

"All About Puberty." *KidsHealth*. Nemours Foundation. October 2015. KidsHealth.org/en/kids/puberty.html.

Anderson, Monica and JingJing Jiang. "Teens, Social Media, and Technology." Pew Research Center. May 31, 2018. PewResearch.org/internet/2018/05/31/teens-social -media-technology-2018.

Bailey, Jacqui and Jan McCafferty. *Sex, Puberty, and All that Stuff*. Hauppauge, NY: Barron's Educational Series, 2004.

"Boys and Puberty." *KidsHealth*. Nemours Foundation. September 2014. KidsHealth.org/en/kids/boys-puberty.html.

Brackett, Marc, Susan E. Rivers, Maria R. Reyes, and Peter Salovey. "Enhancing Academic Performance and Social and Emotional Competence with the RULER Feeling Words Curriculum." *Learning and Individual Differences* 22, no. 2 (April 2012): 218–224. doi.org/10.1016/j.lindif.2010.10.002.

"Child and Adolescent Mental Health." National Institutes of Health. Last modified May 2019. NIMH.NIH.gov/health /topics/child-and-adolescent-mental-health/index.shtml.

"Child Maltreatment Survey." Children's Bureau, Health and Human Services Administration for Children and Families. January 2021. ACF.HHS.gov/cb/data-research/child-maltreatment.

"Coming of Age: Adolescent Health." World Health Organization. Last modified 2021. WHO.int/news-room/spotlight/coming -of-age-adolescent-health.

"Effectiveness of Family Planning Methods." Centers for Disease Control and Prevention. July 2021. CDC.gov/reproductivehealth /unintendedpregnancy/pdf/family-planning-methods-2014.pdf.

"Gender Dysphoria." Mayo Clinic. Accessed July 2021. MayoClinic .org/diseases-conditions/gender-dysphoria/symptoms-causes /syc-20475255.

Holbrook, Calvin. "Male Loneliness: The Ticking Time Bomb That's Killing Men." Happiness.com. Accessed July 2021. Happiness.com/magazine/health-body/male-loneliness -time-bomb-killing-men.

"Internet Safety Tips For Kids." Safe Search Kids. Accessed July 2021. SafeSearchKids.com/internet-safety-tips-for-kids.

"Intersex Fact Sheet." United Nations for LGBT Equality (UNFE). May 2017. UNFE.org/wp-content/uploads/2017/05 /UNFE-Intersex.pdf.

Lenhart, Amanda, Monica Anderson, and Aaron Smith. "Teens, Technology and Romantic Relationships." Pew Research Center. October 1, 2015. PewResearch.org/internet /2015/10/01/teens-technology-and-romantic-relationships.

Madaras, Lynda. The "What's Happening to My Body?" Book For Boys. New York: New Market Press, 2007.

"Male Reproductive System." TeensHealth. Nemours Foundation. Last modified July 2019. KidsHealth.org/en/teens/male-repro.html.

"Media Reference Guide." GLAAD (Gay & Lesbian Alliance Against Defamation). Accessed July 2021. GLAAD.org/reference.

Moore, Susan. "Teenagers in Love." The British Psychological Society. July 2016. ThePsychologist.BPS.org.uk/volume-29 /july/teenagers-love.

Newman, Tim. "Sex and Gender: What is the Difference?" *Medical News Today*. May 11, 2021. MedicalNewsToday.com/articles /232363.

"Physical Development in Boys: What to Expect." American Academy of Pediatrics. May 22, 2015. HealthyChildren.org/English/ages -stages/gradeschool/puberty/Pages/Physical-Development-Boys -What-to-Expect.aspx.

"Porn Literacy." Berkeley University Health Services. Accessed July 2021. UHS.Berkeley.edu/sites/default/files/porn_literacy .pdf.

Robinson, Lawrence and Jeanne Segal. "Bullying and Cyberbullying." HelpGuide. Last modified November 2020. HelpGuide.org /articles/abuse/bullying-and-cyberbullying.htm.

Salter, Michael. "The Problem With a Fight Against Toxic Masculinity." *The Atlantic*. February 27, 2019. TheAtlantic.com /health/archive/2019/02/toxic-masculinity-history/583411.

"Sexual Attraction and Orientation." *TeensHealth*. Nemours Foundation. October 2015. KidsHealth.org/en/teens /sexual-orientation.html.

"Sexual Health." Centers for Disease Control and Prevention. June 2019. CDC.gov/sexualhealth.

"Sexual Health." World Health Organization. Accessed July 2021. WHO.int/health-topics/sexual-health.

"Suicide Statistics." American Foundation for Suicide Prevention. Accessed July 2021. AFSP.org/suicide-statistics.

"Top Signs Boys Are In Puberty." *Amaze*. Accessed July 2021. Amaze.org/video/top-signs-boys-are-in-puberty.

"What Are Wet Dreams?" *TeensHealth*. Nemours Foundation. Last modified October 2019. KidsHealth.org/en/teens/expert -wet-dreams.html.

"What Is Digital Literacy?" *Common Sense Media*. Accessed July 2021. CommonSenseMedia.org/news-and-media-literacy/what-is -digital-literacy.

"What Consent Does—and Doesn't—Look Like." *Love Is Respect*. Accessed July 2021. LoveIsRespect.org/healthy-relationships /what-consent.

"What Consent Looks Like." *RAINN*. Accessed July 2021. RAINN .org/articles/what-is-consent.

"Youth Risk Behavior Surveillance." Centers for Disease Control and Prevention. August 21, 2020. CDC.gov/healthyyouth/data /yrbs/pdf/2019/su6901-H.pdf.

INDEX

A

Abortion, 45–46
Abstinence, 42, 102, 130
Acne, 10
Addiction, 30
Adolescence, defined, xiii
Advocacy, 67–68, 117
Aggression, 29
Allyship, 117–121, 132
Anal sex, 42
Anger, 28
Asexuality, 41

B

Barrier protection, 46, 131
Birth control. *See* Contraception
Bisexuality, 40
Body hair, 8
Body image, xv
Body odor, 8–9, 125
Body positivity, xv–xvi
Boundaries, xvii, 65, 72–73
"Boys will be boys" mentality, 20
Breakups, 88–90, 132

C

Chlamydia, 42–43, 46
Cisgender, 37
Coming out, 127
Comparison to others, 25–26
Compassion, developing, 17–18
Condoms, 44–45, 46, 130–131
Consent
    defined, 13, 91
    in every relationship, 95–97
    FRIES acronym, 92–93
    privacy as a precursor to, 13

Contraception, 44–46, 103, 130–131
Conversations, initiating, xvi–xviii,
    124, 135

D

Dating, 85–90, 128
Disabilities, and sex education,
    131–132
Disrespect, 133
Diverse viewpoints, openness to, 64,
    66–67, 132

E

Egocentrism, 17–18
Ejaculation, 12
Embarrassment, 31
Emergency contraception, 45, 131
Emotional development, 26–31, 32
Emotional intimacy, 75–80
Emotional suppression, 27–28, 32
Erections, 11–12, 15
Estrogen, 6

F

Friendships, 24, 30, 76–77
FRIES acronym, 92–93

G

Gay, 40
Gender
    defined, xiv, 36
    dysphoria, 37
    expression, 36
    identity, 36, 37–38, 127
    stereotypes, 17
Gender neutral language, xiii–xiv
Genitals, 10–12

Gentlemanly behavior, 19, 92
Gonorrhea, 43, 46
Growing pains, 7–8
Growth mindset, 24–25
Growth spurts, 7
Gynecomastia, 8

H

Height, 6–8
Hepatitis B, 43
Herpes simplex virus (HSV), 43
Hormonal contraception, 45, 130–131
Hormones, 6
Human immunodeficiency virus
    (HIV), 44, 46, 131
Human papillomavirus (HPV), 44,
    46, 131
Hydrocele, 12
Hygiene, 9, 15, 125

I

Identity, 35
Intimacy, 75–80
Intrauterine device (IUD), 45, 130

L

Lesbian, 40
LGBTQIA+, xiv, 118, 127
Loneliness, 30

M

Macho mentality, 19
Male, defined, xiii
Masculinity
    positive, 19, 32, 119–120, 129
    toxic, 18–21, 24, 32, 134
Masturbation, 13–14, 126
Maturity, 125
Misogyny, 20, 134
Mood swings, 27, 32
Morning-after pill, 45, 131

N

Nipples, swelling around, 8
Nocturnal emissions, 12, 15

O

Openness, 63–68
Oral sex, 42

P

Pansexuality, 41
Peer pressure, 23, 65
Penis, 10–12
Peyronie's disease, 12
Phimosis, 12
Pornography, 104–109, 128
Positivity, xv–xvi
Privacy, 13–15, 127
Pronouns, 38–39, 47, 133
Puberty
    body hair and odor, 8–9
    defined, xiii
    genital changes, 10–12
    height and weight changes, 6–8
    signs of, 6, 124
    skin changes, 10
    timeline, 6, 15
    voice changes, 9–10
Purpose, 120

Q

Queer, 41
Questions, answering, xviii–xix,
    124–125

R

Relationships
    dating, 85–90, 128
    incorporating consent in, 95–97
    intimacy in, 75–80
    same-sex friendships, 24
    social, 22–23
Respect, 57–62

S

School routines, 65
Self-advocacy, 67
Self-affirmation, 34
Self-awareness, 34, 68
Self-care, 34–35
Semen, 12
Sex
  anal, 42
  defined, xiv, 35
  vs. gender, 37–38
  oral, 42
  positivity, xvi, 21, 98, 101–102, 134
  safer, 98–103
  talking about, xii–xx, 126, 135
  vaginal, 42
Sexting, 112–114
Sexual contact, xiv, 99–100, 127,
    134–135
Sexual health, 41–46, 47
Sexuality, 39–41, 47
Sexually transmitted infections
    (STIs), 42–44, 46, 101, 130–131,
    134–135
Sexual prowess, 21
Sexual violence, 93
Sexual wellness, xiii
Shame, 31
Skin conditions, 10

Social development, 21–26, 32
Social media, 78, 110–115, 129, 133
Sperm cells, 12
Substance abuse, 30
Suicide, 30
Syphilis, 43, 46

T

Testicles, 10
Testicular torsion, 12
Testosterone, 6
Texting, 110–115
THINK acronym, 114–115
Toxic masculinity, 18–21, 24, 32, 134
Transgender, 37, 133
Treatments, for STIs, 46
Trust, 57–62

V

Vaginal sex, 42
Values, 51–56
Virginity, 42
Voice changes, 9–10
Vulnerability, 19, 69–74, 89

W

Weight, 6–8
Wet dreams, 12, 15
Withdrawal method, 130

About the Author

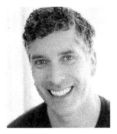

Scott Todnem (he/him) is also the author of *Growing Up Great! The Ultimate Puberty Book for Boys*. Todnem has been teaching Health Education at the middle school level since 2001 and was honored as the 2019 National Health Teacher of the Year. He uses his platforms to promote gender inclusivity, cultural diversity, mental health awareness, suicide prevention, and comprehensive sex education.

Todnem is a nationally recognized presenter and travels to speak about the benefits of quality health education programs. He has organized educational trips to state and national capitals and coached cross-country and track and field for years, developing a passion for running and helping young people lead active lifestyles. Todnem's interest in exercise and weightlifting led the way to his becoming a community fitness leader as co-owner of a strength and conditioning facility for people of all ages.

Todnem enjoys adding to the health class experience by hosting a YouTube channel and a podcast with his students, both of which can be found at LifeIsTheFuture.com. He currently resides in Illinois with his family, where he enjoys reading, record collecting, and weekly movie nights. Additional writing, email newsletters, and other content is available on LifeIsTheFuture.com.